Environmental Health Criteria 45

CAMPHECHLOR

Published under the joint sponsorship of
the United Nations Environment Programme,
the International Labour Organisation,
and the World Health Organization

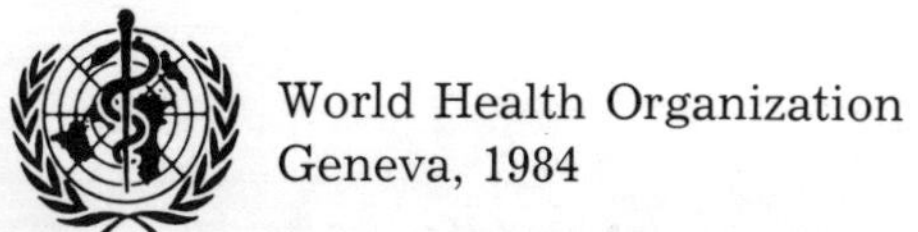

World Health Organization
Geneva, 1984

The **International Programme on Chemical Safety (IPCS)** is a joint venture of the United Nations Environment Programme, the International Labour Organisation, and the World Health Organization. The main objective of the IPCS is to carry out and disseminate evaluations of the effects of chemicals on human health and the quality of the environment. Supporting activities include the development of epidemiological, experimental laboratory, and risk-assessment methods that could produce internationally comparable results, and the development of manpower in the field of toxicology. Other activities carried out by the IPCS include the development of know-how for coping with chemical accidents, coordination of laboratory testing and epidemiological studies, and promotion of research on the mechanisms of the biological action of chemicals.

ISBN 92 4 154185 7

The designations employed and the presentation of the material in this publication do not imply the expression of any opinion whatsoever on the part of the Secretariat of the World Health Organization concerning the legal status of any country, territory, city or area or of its authorities, or concerning the delimitation of its frontiers or boundaries.

The mention of specific companies or of certain manufacturers' products does not imply that they are endorsed or recommended by the World Health Organization in preference to others of a similar nature that are not mentioned. Errors and omissions excepted, the names of proprietary products are distinguished by initial capital letters.

PRINTED IN FINLAND

84/6278 – VAMMALA – 5500

CONTENTS

Page

NOTE TO READERS OF THE CRITERIA DOCUMENTS

While every effort has been made to present information in the criteria documents as accurately as possible without unduly delaying their publication, mistakes might have occurred and are likely to occur in the future. In the interest of all users of the environmental health criteria documents, readers are kindly requested to communicate any errors found to the Manager of the International Programme on Chemical Safety, World Health Organization, Geneva, Switzerland, in order that they may be included in corrigenda, which will appear in subsequent volumes.

In addition, experts in any particular field dealt with in the criteria documents are kindly requested to make available to the WHO Secretariat any important published information that may have inadvertently been omitted and which may change the evaluation of health risks from exposure to the environmental agent under examination, so that the information may be considered in the event of updating and re-evaluation of the conclusions contained in the criteria documents.

* * *

A detailed data profile and a legal file can be obtained from the International Register of Potentially Toxic Chemicals, Palais des Nations, 1211 Geneva 10, Switzerland (Telephone No. 988400 - 985850).

TASK GROUP MEETING ON ENVIRONMENTAL HEALTH CRITERIA FOR ORGANOCHLORINE PESTICIDES OTHER THAN DDT (CHLORDANE, HEPTACHLOR, MIREX, CHLORDECONE, KELEVAN, CAMPHECHLOR)

Members

Dr Z. Adamis, National Institute of Occupational Health, Budapest, Hungary

Dr D.A. Akintonwa, Department of Biochemistry, Faculty of Medicine, University of Calabar, Calabar, Nigeria[a]

Dr R. Goulding, Chairman of the Scientific Sub-committee, UK Pesticides Safety Precautions Scheme, Ministry of Agriculture, Fisheries & Food, London, England (Chairman)

Dr S.K. Kashyap, National Institute of Occupational Health (Indian Council of Medical Research), Meghaninager, Ahmedabad, India

Dr D.C. Villeneuve, Environmental Contaminants Section, Environmental Health Centre, Tunney's Pasture, Ottawa, Ontario, Canada (Rapporteur)

Dr D. Wassermann, Department of Occupational Health, The Hebrew University, Haddassah Medical School, Jerusalem, Israel (Vice-Chairman)

Representatives of Other Organizations

Dr C.J. Calo, European Chemical Industry Ecology and Toxicology Centre (ECETOC)

Mrs M.Th. van der Venne, Commission of the European Communities, Health and Safety Directorate, Luxembourg

Dr D.M. Whitacre, International Group of National Associations of Agrochemical Manufacturers (GIFAP)

Secretariat

Dr M. Gilbert, International Register for Potentially Toxic Chemicals, United Nations Environment Programme, Geneva, Switzerland

---

[a] Unable to attend.

Secretariat (contd).

Mrs B. Goelzer, Division of Noncommunicable Diseases, Office of Occupational Health, World Health Organization, Geneva, Switzerland

Dr Y. Hasegawa, Division of Environmental Health, Environmental Hazards and Food Protection, World Health Organization, Geneva, Switzerland

Dr K.W. Jager, Division of Environmental Health, Internationational Programme on Chemical Safety, World Health Organization, Geneva, Switzerland (*Secretary*)

Mr B. Labarthe, International Register for Potentially Toxic Chemicals, United Nations Environment Programme, Geneva, Switzerland

Dr I.M. Lindquist, International Labour Organisation, Geneva, Switzerland

Dr M. Vandekar, Division of Vector Biology and Control, Pesticides Development and Safe Use Unit, World Health Organization, Geneva, Switzerland

Mr J.D. Wilbourn, Unit of Carcinogen Identification and Evaluation, International Agency for Research on Cancer, Lyons, France

ENVIRONMENTAL HEALTH CRITERIA FOR CAMPHECHLOR

Following the recommendations of the United Nations Conference on the Human Environment held in Stockholm in 1972, and in response to a number of World Health Assembly Resolutions (WHA23.60, WHA24.47, WHA25.58, WHA26.68), and the recommendation of the Governing Council of the United Nations Environment Programme, (UNEP/GC/10, 3 July 1973), a programme on the integrated assessment of the health effects of environmental pollution was initiated in 1973. The programme, known as the WHO Environmental Health Criteria Programme, has been implemented with the support of the Environment Fund of the United Nations Environment Programme. In 1980, the Environmental Health Criteria Programme was incorporated into the International Programme on Chemical Safety (IPCS). The result of the Environmental Health Criteria Programme is a series of criteria documents.

A WHO Task Group on Environmental Health Criteria for Organochlorine Pesticides other than DDT met in Geneva from 28 November to 2 December 1983. Dr K.W. Jager opened the meeting on behalf of the Director-General. The Task Group reviewed and revised the draft criteria document and made an evaluation of the health risks of exposure to camphechlor.

This document is a combination of drafts prepared by Dr D.C. Villeneuve of Canada and Dr S. Dobson of the United Kingdom.

The efforts of all who helped in the preparation and finalization of the document are gratefully acknowledged.

* * *

Partial financial support for the publication of this criteria document was kindly provided by the United States Department of Health and Human Services, through a contract from the National Institute of Environmental Health Sciences, Research Triangle Park, North Carolina, USA - a WHO Collaborating Centre for Environmental Health Effects.

1. SUMMARY AND RECOMMENDATIONS

1.1 Summary

1.1.1 Identity, properties and analytical methods

Camphechlor (toxaphene) ($C_{10}H_{10}Cl_8$ approx.) is an amber, waxy solid consisting of a complex mixture of polychlorinated bicyclic terpenes.

Gas chromatography with electron capture detection is the method of choice for the determination of camphechlor.

1.1.2 Use and sources of exposure

Camphechlor is a non-systemic contact and stomach insecticide with some acaricidal action. It is often used in combination with other pesticides.

The main source of exposure for the general population is the residues of camphechlor in food, but these are generally very low.

1.1.3 Environmental concentrations and exposure

Camphechlor is broken down in the environment by sunlight (ultraviolet radiation), high temperature, and by biodegradation. There are no details on the relative breakdown of the components of the mixture. Camphechlor is readily lost from the soil by evaporation, but, once it penetrates the soil,it is tightly bound to soil particles and very resistent to leaching. Its half-life in soil has been reported to vary from 70 days to 12 years, depending on the type and condition of the soil. In some waters it has been shown to persist for years at concentrations that are toxic for fish.

Camphechlor is rapidly removed from crops by weathering and evaporation.

It is toxic for aquatic species and some terrestrial species and has been shown to bioaccumulate, mainly in aquatic species. It may present a major hazard for aquatic organisms. It also poses a threat to birds.

1.1.4 Kinetics and metabolism

Camphechlor is absorbed following ingestion and inhalation, as well as through the skin. Detailed information is lacking on its metabolism, probably because of its complex composition. Both hydroxylation and dechlorination products have been found as metabolites. Excretion takes place via both urine and faeces.

1.1.5 Studies on experimental animals

Camphechlor is moderately toxic, i.e., the oral LD_{50} values in the rat range from 60 to 120 mg/kg body weight and can on acute oral overexposure give rise to salivation, vomiting, hyperexcitability, convulsions, and death. The lethal dose for man is estimated to be 2 - 7 g. It is an irritant for the skin.

In short-term and long-term studies on animals, hypertrophy of the liver with increased microsomal enzyme activity and histological changes in the liver cells occurs at high dose levels (1000 mg/kg diet), depending on the test conditions and the species tested. Induction of microsomal enzyme activity in the rat has been found at levels of 5 mg or more/kg diet. Hypertrophy of the thyroid and adrenals and degeneration of the tubular epithelium of the kidney have also been reported. At near lethal dosages, excitation of the CNS may occur.

Camphechlor has been shown not to have any effects on reproduction and was not found to be teratogenic. It was mutagenic in *Salmonella typhimurium* but results of a dominant lethal test on mice were negative. It is carcinogenic for both rats and mice.

1.1.6 Effects on man

Several cases of poisoning have been described in man due to contamination of food with camphechlor or to accidental ingestion of camphechlor formulations. Symptomatology consists of gastrointestinal complaints, followed by motor seizures. Some incidents in children were lethal.

Although a survey of a population of workers in a plant manufacturing camphechlor did not reveal any cases of ill-health referable to their employment, some illness has been reported in a few people coming into contact with this chemical. A group of 8 women exposed to camphechlor were reported to have a higher incidence of chromosome abnormalities than the controls. Available epidemiological studies are not adequate to evaluate the carcinogenicity of camphechlor for human beings.

1.2 Recommendations

1. Careful surveillance should be maintained over the future production of camphechlor and the nature and extent of its use.

2. Levels in the environment should continue to be comprehensively monitored.

2. IDENTITY, PHYSICAL AND CHEMICAL PROPERTIES, AND ANALYTICAL METHODS

2.1 Identity

Chemical structure:

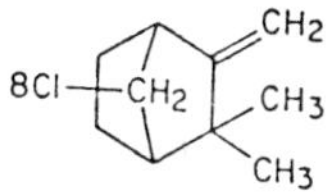

$$8Cl - C_{10}H_{10} \text{ (chlorinated camphene: bicyclic ring with bridging } CH_2\text{, =}CH_2\text{, and two } CH_3\text{)}$$

Molecular formula: $C_{10}H_{10}Cl_8$ (approximately)

CAS chemical name: Toxaphene (a mixture of polychlorinated bicyclic terpenes with chlorinated camphenes predominating)

Trade names: Altox, Chem-Phene M5055, Chlor Chem T-590, Crestoxo, Estonox, Fasco-Terpene, Geniphene, Gy-Phene, Hercules 3956, Huilex, Penphene, Phenacide, Phenatox, Polychlorcamphen, Strobane-T, Toxakil, Toxaphene, Toxon 63

CAS registry number: 8001-35-2

Relative molecular mass: 413.8 (average)

2.2 Physical and Chemical Properties

Camphechlor is an amber, waxy solid (Canada, Department of National Health and Welfare, 1978) with a melting range of 65 - 90 °C. Its vapour pressure is $3.3 \cdot 10^{-5}$ mm Hg at 20 - 25 °C. Camphechlor may dechlorinate in the presence of alkali, sunlight (UV radiation) or at temperatures above 120 °C (Canada, Department of National Health and Welfare, 1978; IARC, 1979). It is soluble in common organic solvents but practically insoluble in water (0.4 - 3.0 mg/litre) (Metcalf, 1976).

The exact chemical structure has not yet been elucidated (von Rumker et al., 1974). The technical product is a complex mixture of chlorinated bicyclic terpenes containing 67 - 69% chlorine by weight (Canada, Department of National Health and Welfare, 1978), which result from the chlorination of pine resins. Camphechlor has been separated into at least 177 C_{10}-polychloro compounds, including Cl_6, Cl_7, Cl_8, Cl_9, and Cl_{10} derivatives, using absorption and gas-liquid chromatography (Casida et al., 1974, Holmstead et al., 1974).

2.3 Analytical Methods

Much difficulty has been encountered in the determination of camphechlor residues due to the fact that camphechlor is not a single compound, but a mixture of over 177 compounds. In addition, it is often used in conjunction with other pesticides, which may cause interference in analytical procedures for camphechlor residues.

Several analytical methods used for the determination of camphechlor in air, water, soil, food, and animal tissues are summarized in Table 1 (IARC, 1979).

Table 1. Methods for the determination of camphechlor

Sample type	Sampling method extraction/clean-up	Analytical method	Limit of detection	Reference
Air				
workplace	trap on cellulose membrane, extract (petroleum ether)	GC/ECD	0.225 - 1.155 mg/m³	NIOSH (1977b)
Water				
fish-tank	extract (acetone-petroleum ether) in a special syphon system, wash resulting water-acetone layer (petroleum ether), bulk petroleum ether fractions, CC	GC/ECD	10 µg/litre	Stalling & Huckins (1976)
Soil	moisten (water), extract (hexane-isopropanol), wash (water)	GC/ECD	0.05 - 0.1 mg/kg	Carey et al. (1976)
Food				
molasses	dilute (water), extract (hexane-isopropanol)	GC/ECD	0.03 mg/kg	Yang et al. (1976)
fruits and vegetables	extract (acetone) in blender, filter, extract (petroleum ether-dichloromethane), wash aqueous phase (dichloromethane), bulk solvent extracts, evaporate to small bulk, add acetone, reduce volume and repeat, CC	GC/ECD		Luke et al. (1975)
Biological tissues	macerate, add anhydrous sodium sulfate, extract (acetone), add water, extract (chloroform) wash (potassium hydroxide solution)	TLC	1 µg	Tewari & Sharma (1977)

CC = column chromatography; GC = gas chromatography; ECD = electron capture detection; TLC = thin-layer chromatography.

3. PRODUCTION AND USES, TRANSPORT AND DISTRIBUTION

3.1 Production and Uses

Camphechlor does not occur naturally in the environment (Canada, Department of National Health and Welfare, 1978). Camphechlor has been in use since 1949 and, in 1975, it was the most heavily-used insecticide in the USA (Pollock & Kilgore, 1980). In 1969, 168 uses for camphechlor were registered in the USA.

Production in the USA has been estimated to range from 22 700 - 40 800 tonnes per year (Canada, Department of National Health and Welfare, 1978). Von Rumker et al. (1974) gave the following annual figures for the USA: total production 34 200 tonnes, of which 8000 tonnes was exported and 26 500 tonnes was used in the USA: 450 tonnes for industrial application and 25 650 tonnes for agricultural use. Estimated consumption in the USA was 9360 tonnes in 1980 and 5400 tonnes in 1982. Since late 1982, use in the USA has been limited to scabies control on cattle and sheep, insect control on pineapples and bananas in the Virgin Islands and Puerto Rico, and for emergency use against army worms and grasshoppers on cotton, corn, and grain. These uses are restricted to certified spray operators wearing protective clothing (IRPTC, 1983a). Registered uses in Canada are minimal and are decreasing.

Camphechlor is a non-systemic contact and stomach insecticide with some acaricidal action. The primary crops on which camphechlor is used are cotton, cereal grains, fruits, nuts, oil seeds, and vegetables. Use on livestock is primarily for the control of ticks and mites. The use of camphechlor on crops has not been a serious problem for bees fertilizing the treated crops (WHO, 1975). Camphechlor is often mixed with other pesticides and appears to act as a solubilizer for insecticides with low solubility. The synergistic properties of camphechlor when used with some other insecticides have been reported (von Rumker et al., 1974). Camphechlor is often applied together with DDT or methyl or ethyl parathion (WHO, 1975).

3.2 Transport and Distribution

3.2.1 Air

The major route of removal of camphechlor from the soil is through evaporation (von Rumker et al., 1974). Although there is little information on the atmospheric transport of camphechlor, it is likely that it may cover hundreds of miles. Camphechlor levels in 75 out of 880 air samples from different parts of the USA ranged between 68 and 2520 ng/m³ (Stanley et al., 1971). Five out of 8 rainwater samples taken in Maryland, USA, contained camphechlor (Munson, 1976).

3.2.2 Water

Accumulation of camphechlor occurs in water in areas where the insecticide is in use and it may be quite persistent. It has been found in water in some lakes, in toxic concentrations, for up to 5 years after fish have been killed (Canada, Department of National Health and Welfare, 1978). Camphechlor was not found in drinking-water supplies in Canada above a detection level of 0.01 mg/litre (Canada, Department of National Health and Welfare, 1978). In the USA, camphechlor concentrations were usually less than 0.001 mg/litre; nevertheless, concentrations as high as 0.065 mg/litre were found in some areas where cotton had been sprayed several months earlier (Bradley et al., 1972). Camphechlor concentrations of up to about 2 g/kg were found in the sediment of a stream that received the effluent of a camphechlor-manufacturing plant (Durant & Reimold, 1972). Camphechlor residues in the range of 7 - 410 ng/litre were also present in all water samples taken before and after treatment by a water treatment plant (Nicholson et al., 1964).

Although the majority of the residues are volatilized, levels in runoff from soil surfaces or treated plants may be substantial (von Rumker et al., 1974).

3.2.3 Soil

As camphechlor is applied topically to livestock and agricultural crops, very little of the pesticide gets mixed into the soil. However, that which penetrates into the soil becomes tightly bound to soil particles and is then highly resistant to leaching (von Rumker et al., 1974). Residues adsorbed on soil particles may be transported via soil erosion and sediment transport. The downward migration of camphechlor in soil is not significant. The results of a study assessing the vertical distribution of camphechlor indicated that, after 3 years, 85 - 90% of the remaining pesticide was in the top 23 cm of the soil (WHO, 1975).

The half-life of camphechlor in soil has been found to vary from 70 days (in moist, sandy soil) to 179 days (in moist clay soil). The half-life in these same soils, if dried, became 136 and 705 days, respectively (WHO, 1975). In another study, involving the mixing of camphechlor with soil, 45% of the original application remained after 14 years (Nash &

Woolson, 1967). Other authors have determined that the half-life of camphechlor in soil ranges from 100 days (LaFleur et al., 1973) up to 6 and 12 years (Alexander, 1965; Nash & Woolson, 1967; Menzie, 1972). The disparity among these findings may be explained by variations in soil type and climates.

No evidence has been found to suggest the existence of conversion products of camphechlor in weathered crop residues (WHO, 1975). However, camphechlor is rapidly removed from crops by weathering and volatilization.

In the USA, the average level of camphechlor in cropland soil is 0.07 mg/kg. A study on 969 soil samples from cropland soils from 43 states and on non-cropland soils from 11 states showed camphechlor residues in only 4.2% of the sites examined, despite the fact that all the major camphechlor-using areas were included in the cropland states surveyed. In the 199 non-cropland soil samples, camphechlor occurred only once (Wiersma et al., 1972a,b,c).

3.2.4 Abiotic degradation

Camphechlor is broken down by sunlight (ultraviolet radiation) and high temperatures. It is also biologically degraded by soil bacteria and fungi, the bacteria utilizing it as a source of carbon (WHO/FAO, 1975). No definitive data have been published on the degradation pathways of the mixture of compounds found in camphechlor (Metcalf, 1976).

4. ENVIRONMENTAL LEVELS AND EXPOSURES

4.1 Environmental Levels

4.1.1 Air

Because the concentrations of camphechlor in ambient air in unsprayed areas are in the ng/m^3 range (IARC, 1979), it seems unlikely that it would cause any health hazard.

4.1.2 Water

Only bodies of water that have been treated with camphechlor for fish control or receive runoff from manufacturing sites or cropland areas treated with camphechlor have been found to contain significant amounts of camphechlor.

The lower limit of detection of camphechlor by taste is approximately 5 µg/litre. Water treated with activated carbon (a method used to clear water bodies of accidental camphechlor spills) is effectively free of camphechlor (WHO, 1975). No damage to man resulting from camphechlor residues in water has been reported.

4.1.3 Food

Camphechlor bioaccumulates and builds up in food chains, but not to the same extent as some other highly persistent chlorinated hydrocarbons (von Rumker et al., 1974). For the most part, camphechlor levels in food seem to be below the national tolerances (WHO, 1975), which range from 2 - 7 mg/kg in Australia, Canada, and the USA, and are as low as 0.4 mg/kg in the Federal Republic of Germany and the Netherlands (WHO, 1975).

Camphechlor was evaluated by the Joint Meeting on Pesticide Residues (JMPR) in 1968 and 1973 (FAO/WHO, 1969, 1974). In 1968, no recommendations were made because of the many unresolved questions. In 1973, the meeting concluded that it could not establish an ADI for a material that varied in composition according to the method of manufacture.

Because camphechlor is not a systemic insecticide, the residues are more or less confined to the plant surfaces (WHO, 1975). Camphechlor residues generally occur in agricultural crops as well as in meat from domestic livestock and fish. Thirty-one days following an application of camphechlor to alfalfa, 72.9% of the compound had been lost. Long-term losses depended on the quantity applied, the formulation, and the application route. The greatest residue was left from oily solutions, followed by water emulsions and by dusts (Pollock & Kilgore, 1978). Camphechlor residues on growing leafy crops have a half-life of 5 - 10 days. On alfalfa and clover, the half-life is in the range of 9 - 13 days. The residue level is controlled by time of application, dosage rate, and appropriate pre-slaughter or pre-harvest intervals (WHO, 1975).

Fruits and vegetables have been found to contain camphechlor residues; the highest concentrations were found in spinach (FAO/WHO, 1969). In studies conducted during 1964-67, the average levels of camphechlor residues found in leaf and stem vegetables was 0.18 mg/kg and that in processed foods 0.45 mg/kg. Generally, levels of camphechlor in all foods were low. In 1964-66, camphechlor residues were detected in 30, 8, and 2% of the cottonseed, soybean, and peanut oil samples listed, respectively (Pollock & Kilgore, 1978). Heat processing of fruits and vegetables was found to reduce levels of camphechlor residues (WHO, 1975). Sugar beet, sampled in the USA in the autumn of 1970, showed camphechlor residues of 0 - 0.34 mg/kg (Yang et al., 1976). It has been demonstrated that peeling, abrasive peeling, and washing removes most of the camphechlor residues present on fruits and vegetables. The addition of 0.1% synthetic detergent or 1.0% neutral soap to the washing water increases the amount of the pesticide removed (WHO, 1975).

Honey produced by bees exposed to ^{36}Cl-camphechlor contained less than 0.01 mg camphechlor/kg (WHO, 1975).

Because livestock is treated with camphechlor to remove external insects and because some feeds are contaminated with camphechlor, camphechlor residues are found in meat and poultry. The residues in meat can be significantly reduced by trimming excess fat (the primary storage site for camphechlor) and also by cooking at temperatures sufficient to render out the fat (WHO, 1975). In animals, the level of storage of camphechlor is lower and its elimination more rapid than with most other chlorinated hydrocarbons (FAO/WHO, 1974), hence residues in poultry and meat are very low (WHO, 1975). In general, the level stored in the fat of sheep and cattle is 25 - 50% of the level in the feed. This concentration is less in hogs, probably because of a greater fat content (FAO/WHO, 1969).

Camphechlor has been detected in the milk from cows sprayed or fed this insecticide (Clayborn et al., 1963; Canada, Department of National Health and Welfare, 1978). The ratio of camphechlor concentration in feed to that in milk is approximately 100:1. Build-up in milk quickly fades when exposure to camphechlor is discontinued (WHO, 1975). Residues of camphechlor in milk, due to feed containing 5 - 20 mg camphechlor/kg, plateaued after 28 days. Residues in milk, due to feed containing 2.5 mg camphechlor/kg, plateaued by the 9th day. Milk contained 0.11 and 0.18 mg camphechlor residues/litre when feed contained 10 and 20 mg/kg, respectively. The residues in milk fell off sharply, 4 days after camphechlor was absent from the diet and were negligible by the 14th day (Zweig et al., 1963). In the USA, camphechlor was detected in only 5 out of 7265 meat samples and 2 out of 5504 poultry samples (Guyer et al., 1971).

In a study carried out by the Department of National Health and Welfare, Canada, between 1969 and 1971, no detectable levels (at the ppb level) of camphechlor were found in any of the several hundred food items analysed (Smith, 1971; Smith et al., 1972, 1973), while, in another study carried out by the Department of National Health and Welfare, Canada, between 1974 and 1975, unspecified amounts of camphechlor were found in 0.6% of the food items tested (Coffin & McLeod, 1975); thus, the incidence was very low.

In the USA, between 1971 and 1972, among a total of 420 samples of food analysed, only one was found to contain camphechlor (Manske & Johnson, 1975). In a study conducted in the USA during the period of 1964-69, residues of camphechlor were found to be the 6th most frequent in occurrence of all pesticides in processed foods. However, levels were so low that few, if any, exceeded the 7 mg/kg tolerance level (WHO, 1975).

4.1.4 Miscellaneous sources

Camphechlor residues have also been found in non-food items. Camphechlor residues in chewing tobacco, smoking tobacco, snuff, cigarettes, and cigars in the USA were found to have decreased over the period 1971-73. The average concentration in cigarettes decreased from 3.3 to 1.4 mg/kg (Domanski et al., 1974). In 1972, examination showed that 6 brands of cigars purchased in 5 cities in the USA contained camphechlor residues ranging from 0.5 to 3.42 mg/kg (Domanski & Guthrie, 1974), while results of a study conducted in 1970 (Domanski & Sheets, 1973), showed camphechlor residues in tobacco in the USA to be as high as 12 mg/kg.

4.1.5 Wildlife

Residues of camphechlor were found in 53% of samples of fish and invertebrates taken from waters near cotton-producing areas along the Guatemalan Pacific Coast (Keiser et al., 1973). No changes in camphechlor levels were observed when fish containing 5 - 10 mg/kg camphechlor were boiled or fried (Terriere & Ingalsbe, 1953).

Residues have been found infrequently and at low levels in non-aquatic wildlife (Pollock & Kilgore, 1978).

4.2 General Population Exposure

Camphechlor exposure of the general population can result from residues in food.

4.3 Occupational Exposure

Results of a study conducted in camphechlor-manufacturing plants in the USSR showed camphechlor levels 5 - 6 times the permissible limit of 0.2 mg/m^3. After a work shift, levels of 30 - 1000 mg/m^2 were found on the uncovered skin of workers, while levels on covered areas ranged up to 40 mg/m^2 (Ashirova, 1971). However, no adverse effects of this occupational exposure have been reported. Although camphechlor was used extensively during the 1960s in agricultural and public health programmes in Alberta, analyses of human tissue from 50 autopsies at the University Hospital in Edmonton in 1967-68 did not reveal camphechlor in any of the 217 tissues examined (Kadis et al., 1970).

5. KINETICS AND METABOLISM

5.1 Human Studies

In a 9-month-old child, poisoned with a 2:1 mixture of camphechlor and DDT, death occurred after convulsions and respiratory failure. Ratios of camphechlor:DDT in the brain and liver were 10:1 and, in the kidney, 3:1 (Haun & Cueto, 1967). No significant levels of camphechlor were found in the skin and subcutaneous tissue taken from 68 children, who died in the perinatal period, in 13 cities in the USA (Zavon et al., 1969).

5.2 Animal Studies

The metabolism of camphechlor has been an area of little research, because of difficulties in detecting a complex and multicomponent substance. However, a few such studies have been published.

About 37% of a single oral dose of technical grade ^{36}Cl-camphechlor, administered to rats at 20 mg/kg body weight, was eliminated in the faeces; 15% was excreted in the urine in 9 days during the same period (Crowder & Dindal, 1974). Rats were dosed orally with solutions containing either ^{36}Cl-camphechlor, ^{36}Cl-camphechlor fractions, or ^{14}C-camphechlor. Urine and faeces samples were collected for 14 days (Ohsawa et al., 1975). The rats excreted (combined urine and methanol extract of faeces) 76% of the ^{36}Cl-camphechlor, 57% of the ^{14}C-camphechlor, and 69 - 94% of the ^{36}Cl-camphechlor fractions. Very little of the material was excreted unmetabolized and the camphechlor had undergone dechlorination.

A dose-related increase in the excretion of camphechlor in the milk of cows, fed diets containing camphechlor at 2.5 - 20 mg/kg, was reported (Zweig et al., 1963). Results of *in vitro* studies, using rat liver homogenates, showed that isolated camphechlor fractions were metabolized to hydroxylated compounds, in addition to dechlorinated products (Chandurkar & Matsumura, 1979). However, the precise chemical structures of these metabolites were not unequivocally identified. Pollack & Kilgore (1976) dosed rats orally with ^{14}C-camphechlor and reported a cumulative elimination of 58% of the dose in the urine and faeces. Increased amounts of polar "activity" and a small increase in non-polar fractions were found in the fat.

6. STUDIES ON EXPERIMENTAL ANIMALS

6.1 Single Exposures

Camphechlor is absorbed through the skin, respiratory tract, and the intestinal tract (FAO/WHO, 1969; Gleason et al., 1969; Gosselin et al., 1976).

The principal toxic manifestations noted in animals exposed to a single dose of camphechlor consist of salivation, vomiting, reflex excitability, and convulsions terminating in respiratory failure (Taylor et al., 1979). Typical LD_{50} values for a variety of animals are given in Table 2. The influence of the solvent on camphechlor uptake can be seen from the wide range of LD_{50}s in this table.

Table 2. The acute toxicity of camphechlor in several animal studies

Species	Route	Vehicle	LD_{50} (mg/kg)	References
Rat	oral	peanut oil	80 - 90	Gaines (1969)
Rat	dermal	xylene	780 - 1075	Gaines (1969)
Rat	oral	corn oil	60	US EPA (1976a)
Rat	oral	kerosene	120	US EPA (1976a)
Mouse	oral	corn oil	112	US EPA (1976a)
Dog	oral	corn oil	49	US EPA (1976a)
Dog	oral	kerosene	over 250	US EPA (1976a)
Guinea-pig	oral	kerosene	365	US EPA (1976a)
Cat	oral	peanut oil	25 - 40	US EPA (1976a)
Rabbit	oral	peanut oil	75 - 100	US EPA (1976a)
Rabbit	oral	kerosene	250 - 500	US EPA (1976a)
Rabbit	dermal	dust	over 4000	US EPA (1976a)
Rabbit	dermal	peanut oil	over 250	US EPA (1976a)
Rabbit	dermal	wettable powder (suspension in water)	1025 - 1075	Johnston & Eden (1953)
Cattle	oral	grain	144	US EPA (1976a)
Goat	oral	xylene	200	US EPA (1976a)
Sheep	oral	xylene	200	US EPA (1976a)

The acute toxicity of camphechlor in rats is increased at least 3-fold by protein deficiency (Gleason et al., 1969). The lethal oral dose for an adult man is estimated to be 2 - 7 g (Conley, 1952).

6.2 Short-Term Exposures

Rats were fed camphechlor at levels of 0.2 - 50 mg/kg diet, for up to 13 weeks (Kinoshita et al., 1966). Camphechlor was observed to induce microsomal enzyme activity at levels of 5.0 mg/kg and higher.

Camphechlor did not induce any effects on the physical appearance, gross pathology, weight gain, or liver cell histology of albino rats fed 2.33 - 189 mg/kg diet, for up to 12 weeks (Clapp et al., 1971).

Camphechlor, when fed to rats for 7 days at 25 mg/kg diet, caused an increase in the metabolism of estrone and inhibited the increase in uterine weight produced by this compound (Welch et al., 1971).

Studies on pregnant albino rats showed that daily oral administration of camphechlor for up to 20 days resulted in interconnected structural and enzymic changes in the cerebral cortex (Badaeva, 1976).

Rats were dosed once, orally, with 120 mg camphechlor/kg body weight and monitored for up to 15 days (Peakall, 1976). Liver weight and microsomal enzyme activity were increased after 5 and 15 days, respectively. In another study in the same report, rats were administered camphechlor at 2.4 mg/kg body weight per day and killed at 1, 3, and 6 months. Liver weight and microsomal enzyme activity increased at all time intervals, but plasma testosterone levels were not affected.

Administration to rats of a single oral dose of 120 mg/kg body weight, as well as a daily dose of 2.4 mg/kg body weight, for 1 or 3 months, produced a disturbance in catecholamine metabolism (Kuzminskaya & Ivanitski, 1979).

Adult male rats were fed diets containing 0, 50, 100, 150, and 200 mg camphechlor/kg for 14 days (Trottman & Desaiah, 1980). No changes were observed in body weight gain, food consumption, brain, kidney, heart, or testes weights; liver weight was increased at 200 mg/kg and thymus weight decreased at 150 and 200 mg/kg. Increased hydroxylation of aniline was observed at all dose levels.

Administration of 5, 50, or 500 mg camphechlor/kg diet to quail for up to 4 months produced hypertrophy of the thyroid with increased uptake of ^{131}I and adrenal hypertrophy (Hurst et al., 1974).

Feeding of camphechlor in the diet at 5, 50, or 100 mg/kg to chickens for 31 weeks induced sternal deformation and nephrosis (Bush et al., 1977). Occasional keel deformation, involving cartilaginous tissue as well as an apparent increase in the growth of cartilage, was found in birds fed 0.50 mg camphechlor/kg.

Camphechlor was administered in capsules at a daily dose of 4 mg/kg body weight to 2 dogs for 44 days and to 2 other dogs for 106 days. Occasional manifestations of acute toxicity (CNS stimulation) occurred for a short time after administration. There were no significant changes in body weight, blood picture, or gross appearance of organs. Histological examination of many organs revealed some damage to the kidney (degeneration of the tubular epithelium) and to the liver (generalized hydropic degenerative changes, but no destruction of the cells). Liver glycogen levels were normal (Lackey, 1949).

6.3 Long-Term Exposures

Four groups, each of 40 rats (20 males and 20 females), were fed camphechlor in the diet at 10, 100, 1000, and 1500 mg/kg. Effects were determined through gross observation, mortality rates, body weight, blood tests, liver weight, liver to body-weight ratio, gross autopsy, and histological examination of the tissues. After 7 1/2 - 10 months of feeding, some of the rats fed 1500 mg/kg and a few of the rats fed 1000 mg/kg suffered occasional convulsions. The body weight gain of the rats fed the highest feeding level (1500 mg/kg) for the first 20 weeks was less than that in the controls, probably because of decreased food intake through unpalatability of the diet. As the rats became accustomed to the diet, growth rate was essentially the same as that of the controls. There were no significant effects on mortality rate or on the haematopoietic system. The liver weight and liver to body weight ratio was significantly increased only in the 1000 and 1500 mg/kg groups. Liver changes consisted of swelling, cellular hypertrophy, and proliferation of smooth endoplasmic reticulum with cytoplasmic margination in the centrilobular hepatic cells. These changes occurred to a moderate extent in the 1500 mg/kg group and to a slight extent in the 1000 mg/kg group (Treon et al., unpublished data, 1952).

Six male and 6 female rats per group were fed 50 or 200 mg camphechlor/kg diet for up to 9 months (Ortega et al., 1957). There were no clinical signs of toxicity and no effects on body weight gain, food intake, or liver weights. No histological changes were seen in the kidney or spleen. Three out of 12 rats fed 50 mg/kg diet for 9 months showed histological changes in the liver consisting of centrilobular cell hypertrophy, peripheral migration of basophilic granulation, and the presence of liposphere inclusion bodies. Six of the 12 rats fed 200 mg/kg showed liver changes.

Groups of rats were fed camphechlor in the diet at 25, 100, and 400 mg/kg for their lifetime (Fitzhugh & Nelson, 1951). The only organ that showed significant histological changes was the liver and these occurred at the 100 mg/kg and 400 mg/kg levels. There was centrilobular hepatic cell enlargement with increased oxyphilia and peripheral margination of basophilic granules. The effects at the various feeding levels were summarized by Lehman (1952b), as follows: 400 mg/kg, liver enlargement; 100 mg/kg, no gross effects, but tissue damage occurred; and 25 mg/kg, no tissue damage.

Camphechlor dissolved in maize oil, in gelatin capsules, was administered daily, for 5 days per week, to dogs. A dose of 25 mg/kg body weight was fatal. Two dogs were administered 10 mg/kg (equivalent to 400 mg/kg diet); one dog died after 33 days, but the other lived and was sacrificed after 3 1/2 years. Four dogs were administered 5 mg/kg; all survived and were sacrificed after almost 4 years. No information on the pathological findings was reported (Lehman, 1952b).

Camphechlor was fed daily (6 days per week) for 2 years to 3 male and 5 female dogs, beginning when the animals were approximately 4 months old. Camphechlor was added to the diet, including their drinking liquids, at levels of 10 and 50 mg/kg. The dogs received a daily dose of 0.60 - 1.47 mg/kg or 3.12 - 6.56 mg/kg (equivalent to approximately 40 or 200 mg/kg on a dry diet basis). Gross behaviour, body weight, mortality, peripheral circulating blood elements, gross pathology, organ to body weight ratios, and histopathology were recorded (Treon et al., unpublished data, 1952). There were no effects on behaviour, body weight, mortality, or blood elements, but there were increases in the liver weights, liver to body weight ratios, and moderate liver degeneration at the higher dose level (200 mg/kg). At the lower dose level (40 mg/kg), 1 out of 3 dogs was reported to have slight liver enlargement and slight granularity and vacuolization of the cytoplasm. Re-examination of the sections of these animals failed to confirm any difference from control animals. All other tissues were normal at both feeding levels (Brock & Calandra, 1964).[a]

Groups of dogs, comprising 6 male and 6 females, were fed camphechlor at dietary levels of 5, 10, or 20 mg/kg together with control groups. Two male and 2 female animals were sacrificed after 6, 12, and 24 months. None of the feeding levels produced any changes in organ weights, gross or

---

[a] Brock, D. & Calandra, J.C. (1964) Re-evaluation of microscopic sections from chronic oral toxaphene study, Industrial Bio-Test Laboratories, Inc., unpublished report.

histological examination, or any of the clinical or organ function tests, at any time (Industrial Bio-Test Laboratories Inc., unpublished data, 1965)[a].

Two adult female monkeys were given camphechlor in their food, 6 days per week, at a daily dose of 0.64 - 0.78 mg/kg for 2 years. A third animal served as a control. There were no signs of intoxication and no evidence of tissue or organ damage as evaluated by growth rate, ratios of liver to body weight, spleen to body weight, or histological examination of the tissues (Treon et al, unpublished data, 1952).

6.4 Dermal Toxicity

The acute LD_{50} for rabbits exposed dermally to camphechlor in the dry form was > 4000 mg/kg body weight (Lehman, 1952a). The animals showed only moderate skin irritation and systemic effects were characterized by hyperexcitability but no deaths occurred. The animals recovered in 5 or 6 days. The 90-day dermal LD_{50} has been estimated to be approximately 40 mg/kg body weight for rabbits (Lehman, 1952a).

A review of the effects of camphechlor on livestock revealed that cattle, sheep, and hogs can tolerate repeated applications of solutions containing less than 2% camphechlor (Penumarthy et al., 1976). However, dips containing 2.5% camphechlor emulsion caused toxicosis in cattle.

6.5 Reproduction Studies

A 3-generation, 6-litter reproduction study was conducted with camphechlor. Groups of weanling rats were fed 25 mg/kg diet and 100 mg/kg diet for 79 days before mating. All the animals continued on their respective dietary concentration of camphechlor during mating, gestation, and weaning during 2 generations, or for a period of 36 - 39 weeks. Weanlings from the second litter were selected as parents for the second generation and continued on their respective diets until after weaning of a second litter. A third generation was selected in the same manner. Complete gross and histological examination was performed on all three parental generations after 36 weeks of camphechlor administration. The only pathological changes found were slight alterations in the livers of the 100 mg/kg group, similar to the changes seen in long-term studies. Reproductive performance, fertility, and

---

[a] Industrial Bio-Test Laboratories Inc. (1965) Two-year chronic oral toxicity of toxaphene in beagle dogs (Unpublished report).

lactation were normal. The progeny was viable and normal in size and anatomical structure. Findings among all test animals, 3 parental generations and 6 litters of progeny, were comparable to those in control animals for all variables (Kennedy et al., 1973).

Groups of mice (4 males and 14 females per group) were fed camphechlor in the diet at levels of 0 and 25 mg/kg in a 5-generation, 2 litter-per-generation, reproduction study. No effects were noted on any of the reproduction parameters measured (Keplinger et al., 1970).

Camphechlor in a corn-oil carrier was injected into fertile hen eggs. It did not cause any reduction in hatchability, even at the highest dose used, 1.5 mg/egg (Smith et al., 1970). In another study, white leghorn hens were fed camphechlor at 0, 10, and 100 mg/kg diet (Arscott et al., 1976). Except for a slight decrease in egg production, no adverse effects were observed on fertility, hatchability, or survival of progeny.

6.6 Mutagenicity

Camphechlor did not induce dominant lethal mutations in mice (Epstein et al., 1972). When males were injected with 36 and 180 mg/kg body weight ip and bred with untreated females during 8 weeks, the frequencies of early fetal deaths and preimplantation losses were normal. Negative results were also obtained in animals treated orally for 5 successive days with 40 or 80 mg/kg body weight. In an *in vitro* test to determine breakage of DNA in bacteria, camphechlor did not induce breaks at a significantly higher rate than that occurring in controls (Griffin & Hill, 1978). Camphechlor was mutagenic in a test using *Salmonella typhimurium* without requiring activation by liver homogenate (Hooper et al., 1979).

6.7 Teratogenicity

Camphechlor was administered to mice and rats on days 7 - 16 of gestation by oral intubation at levels of 15 - 35 mg/kg body weight per day (Chernoff & Carver, 1976). The highest dose produced marked maternal mortality in rats and mice and an increase in encephaloceles among offspring of mice. Fetal mortality was slightly increased in mice at all dose levels. Small decreases in fetal body weight and in the number of sternal and caudal ossification centres were observed in rats, mostly in the 25 mg/kg dosage group (Chernoff & Carver, 1976).

6.8 Carcinogenicity

A bioassay of technical grade camphechlor was conducted in mice and rats by administering the test chemical in the feed (NCI, 1979b). Groups of 50 mice of each sex were given time-weighted average doses of 99 or 198 mg/kg diet for 90 - 91 weeks. There was a dose-related decrease in survival in male mice and a decrease in survival in high-dose females. The incidence of hepatocellular carcinomas was dose-related in both males and females. The statistical significance was maintained when the incidence of hepatocellular carcinomas was combined with that of hyperplastic nodules of the liver. It was concluded that, under the conditions of the assay, camphechlor was carcinogenic in male and female B6C3F1 mice.

Fifty rats of each sex were administered camphechlor in their diets at time-weighted average doses of 556 and 1112 mg/kg for male rats, and 540 and 1080 mg/kg for females; the study lasted for 108 - 110 weeks. There were no dose-related effects on survival rates; clinical signs of toxicity in rats included generalized body tremors at week 53 in the high-dose males and females and later, leg paralysis, ataxia, epistaxis, haematuria, and vaginal bleeding. Abdominal distention, diarrhoea, dyspnoea, and rough haircoats were common to both dose groups. At the high dose, 26% (9/35) and at the low-dose, 17% (7/41) of male rats developed follicular-cell carcinoma or adenoma of the thyroid. In the high-dose, female rat group, 17% (7/42) developed thyroid tumours and in the low-dose group only 2%. On the basis of the findings in the above study, it was concluded that the results "suggest carcinogenicity of camphechlor for the thyroid of male and female Osborne-Mendel rats" (NCI, 1979b).

6.9 Other Studies

Camphechlor has also been shown to increase the activity of gluconeogenic enzymes in the rat (Desaiah et al., 1979), alter mitochondrial electron transport *in vitro* (Pardino et al., 1971), and inhibit ATPase activity *in vitro* (Yap et al., 1975) and *in vivo* (Fattah & Crowder, 1980).

Protein deficiency was shown to increase the acute toxicity of camphechlor, 3 to 4-fold (Boyd, 1972b).

7. EFFECTS ON MAN: EPIDEMIOLOGICAL AND CLINICAL STUDIES

7.1 Poisoning Incidents

McGee et al. (1952) described 10 cases of poisoning with 3 deaths; the victims ranged in age from 17 months to 49 years. All ingested camphechlor accidentally either in the form of the insecticide, as in the case of the children, or as camphechlor-polluted food, in the adults. Four of the cases were children aged 17 months to 4 years, of whom three died. All the adults survived. The onset of illness in all but one was characterized by a major motor seizure; the latter had only gastrointestinal complaints. The 3 deaths occurred within a matter of several hours and those who recovered did so in 24 h.

Another poisoning incident involved a 16-month-old child who ingested a material presumed to be camphechlor (Pollock, 1953). Death was preceded by respiratory depression and convulsions.

Another child's death due to camphechlor poisoning was reported in 1967 (Haun & Cueto, 1967). In this case, a 9-month-old girl had been playing with a dust containing 13.8% camphechlor and 7.04% DDT, which was found on her skin and in her mouth. Convulsions, respiratory arrest, and death followed. Cerebral oedema was found at autopsy.

7.2 Occupational Exposure

Two workers involved in harvesting cotton that had been sprayed with camphechlor developed dyspnoea and reduced pulmonary function and were found to have miliary opacities distributed over their lung fields (Warraki, 1963).

Eight women working in an area that had been sprayed with camphechlor at the rate of 2 kg/ha were reported to have a higher incidence of chromosome aberrations (acentric fragments and chromatid exchanges) in cultured lymphocytes (13.1%) than control individuals (1.6%) (Samosh, 1974).

In a review of the chronic toxicity of organochlorine pesticides in man (Deichmann, 1973), a survey of 137 workers involved in the manufacture of camphechlor was reported. The average length of exposure was 3.7 years, but some workers were exposed for as long as 18 years. Physical examinations conducted annually on these people failed to reveal any "adverse effects that could be associated with camphechlor exposure".

An instance was reported where a rancher, who dusted his sheep with a mixture of 5% camphechlor and 1% lindane, demonstrated resistance to the hypothrombinemic effect of warfarin (Jeffery et al., 1976). This effect was attributed to the enzyme-inducing properties of camphechlor, which led to increased metabolism of warfarin.

Two cases of acute aplastic anaemia associated with dermal exposure to camphechlor-lindane mixtures, have been reported. One of these cases terminated in death due to acute myelomonocytic leukaemia (US EPA, 1976a).

In a survey of 199 employees, who worked or had worked with camphechlor between 1949 and 1977, with exposures ranging from 6 months to 26 years (mean 5.23 years), 20 employees died, 1 with cancer of colon; none of these deaths appeared to be related to exposure to camphechlor (US EPA, 1978).

7.3 Controlled Human Studies

Twenty-five human volunteers were exposed to an aerosol of camphechlor in a closed chamber, for 30 min per day, on 10 consecutive days (Shelanski, unpublished data, 1947). After 3 weeks, they received the same exposure on 3 consecutive days. Assuming a retention of 50% of the inhaled camphechlor, each individual absorbed 75 mg camphechlor per day or approximately 1 mg/kg body weight per day. Physical examinations and blood and urine tests did not reveal any abnormalities.

8. EFFECTS ON ORGANISMS IN THE ENVIRONMENT

8.1. Aquatic Organisms

8.1.1 Aquatic invertebrates

The toxicity of camphechlor for aquatic invertebrates is very variable (Tables 3 and 4). Needham (1966) measured levels of mortality at different concentrations of camphechlor for 14 genera of invertebrates and determined the level that each could tolerate for 24 h without any deaths. These are tabulated in Table 5. Tolerance varied from 1 mg/litre for a leech to 10 µg/litre for Haliplus sp. Values for molluscs ranged from 20 µg/litre for the oyster to 460 mg/litre for the mactrid clam in 96-h tests, and for crustacea from 54 ng/litre for a stage I zoeal larva of Sesarma to 290 µg/litre for a stage III zoeal larva of Rhithropanopeus, also in 96-h tests. Resistance to camphechlor may develop. The 24-h LD_{50} for fresh water shrimp taken from an area that had been regularly treated for cotton pests was 10 times that of shrimp taken from a wildlife reserve (Naqvi & Ferguson, 1970). Similarly, cyclopoid copepods from a pesticide-contaminated area had a higher tolerance for camphechlor than cyclopoids from a pesticide-free area (Naqvi & Ferguson, 1968).

The only well-documented sublethal effects on invertebrates are found in oysters. Yearling oysters showed a marked inhibition in shell deposition after a 24-h exposure to 60% camphechlor at 100 µg/litre (Butler et al., 1962). Mature oysters showed reduced activity, as measured by shell opening movements, during 4 weeks exposure to camphechlor at 100 µg/litre.

8.1.2 Fish

A series of studies on fathead minnows, brook trout, and channel catfish (Mayer et al., 1975; Mehrle & Mayer, 1975a,b; Mayer & Mehrle, 1976) document the "broken-back syndrome" in response to camphechlor concentrations ranging from 55 to 621 µg/litre. Fish showed increased levels of calcium but decreased levels of collagen in the backbone; phosphorus levels were unaffected. The backbone became more brittle and sub-lethal electric shock led to multiple fracture at all dose levels. In addition to changes in the calcium/collagen ratio, there was a reduction in the amino acids: alanine, valine, leucine, isoleucine, lysine, phenylalanine, and hydroxyproline in bone collagen. Hydroxyproline was also reduced in skin. Because of the importance of this particular amino acid in collagen formation, it is postulated that camphechlor may

Table 3. Toxicity of camphechlor for aquatic invertebrates[a]

Organism	Temperature (°C)	Size (mm)	End point	Parameter	Concentration (μg/litre)	Reference
American oyster (*Crassostrea virginica*)	27-29		shell growth	96-h EC_{50}	16	Schimmel et al. (1977)
crayfish (*Procambarus acutus*)	from clean area	11.8-14.6	no response to stimuli	48-h EC_{50}	60.7	Albaugh (1972)
	from cotton field	11.8-14.6	no response to stimuli	48-h EC_{50}	90.2	Albaugh (1972)
Daphnia pulex first instar	15.5		immobilisation	48-h EC_{50}	15	Sanders & Cope (1966)
pink shrimp, nauplius (*Penaeus duorarum*)				96-h LC_{50}	2.2	Courtenay & Roberts (1973)
pink shrimp, adult	24.5-26			96-h LC_{50}	1.4 (1.1-1.8)	Schimmel et al. (1977)
drift line crab (*Sesarma cinereum*) stage I zoeal	25			96-h LC_{50}	0.054	Courtenay & Roberts (1973)

[a] A more comprehensive table listing different conditions and exposure times is available on request from IRPTC, Geneva.

Table 4. Toxicity of camphechlor for aquatic organisms

Organism	Stat /flow	Temp (°C)	pH	Size	Alk (mg/litre)	End point	Parameter	Concentration (μg/litre)	Reference
Goldfish (*Carassius auratus*)	stat	25	7.4	1-2 g 38-64 mm	18		96-h LC_{50}	5.6	Henderson et al. (1959)
Bluegill (*Lepomis macrochirus*)	stat	18	7.1	0.6-1.7 g	35		96-h LC_{50}	21 (14-30)	Macek & McAllister (1970
Fathead minnow (*Pimephales promelas*)	stat	12.7	7.1	0.6-1.5 g	35		96-h LC_{50}	3.2 (2.8-3.7)	Macek et al. (1969)
	stat	18	7.1	0.6-1.7 g	35		96-h LC_{50}	14 (9-22)	Macek & McAllister (1970)
Sheepshead minnow (*Cyprinodon variegatus*)	flow	27-29.5			21[a] 25.5		96-h LC_{50}	1.1 (0.9-1.4)	Schimmel et al. (1977)
Mosquito fish (*Gambusia affinis*)	flow	25-26	7.8	0.28 g	28[a]	sensitive	36-h LC_{50}	1	Burke & Ferguson (1969)
	flow	25-26	7.8	0.28 g	28[a]	insensitive	36-h LC_{50}	200	Burke & Ferguson (1969)

Table 4 (contd).

Organism	Stat /flow	Temp (°C)	pH	Size	Alk (mg/litre)	End point	Parameter	Concentration (µg/litre)	Reference
Spot, 1 month (*Leiostomus xanthurus*)	flow	11-28		20 mm	21[b] 28[b]		144-h LC_{50}	0.5	Lowe (1964)
Rainbow trout (*Salmo gairdneri*)		7.2 18.3					96-h LC_{50} 96-h LC_{50}	5.4 1.8	Cope (1965) Cope (1965)
Longnose killifish, juv. (*Fundulus similis*)	flow	28.5-31.5		32-51 mm	10[b] 20[b]		28-day LC_{50}	0.9	Schimmel et al. (1977)
Toad (*Bufo woodhousi*)							48-h LC_{50}	290	Guyer et al. (1971)

[a] Hardness mg/litre.
[b] Salinity °/oo.

Table 5. Concentrations of camphechlor tolerated by invertebrates[a]

Organism	Concentration for zero mortality (μg/litre)	Next higher[b] concentration tested (μg/litre)
Hirudinea	1000	
Gammarus sp.	100	200 (61%)
Hydracarina	1000	
Callibaetis sp.	150	300 (29%)
Aeshna sp.	200	275 (16%)
Lestes sp.	450	500 (19%)
Notonecta sp.	275	300 (29%)
Signara sp.	50	75 (40%)
Limephilus sp.	500	550 (51%)
Haliplus sp.	10	40 (55%)
Hydroporus sp.	60	100 (27%)
Dytiscus sp.	15	50 (24%)
Eyrinus sp.	65	100 (22%)
Lymnara sp.	700	

[a] From: Needham (1966).
[b] Value in parentheses is percentage mortality found at the next higher concentration tested above that giving zero mortality.

reduce the wound-healing capacity in fish. Camphechlor, at concentrations as low as 68 μg/litre, inhibited collagen synthesis (monitored by hydroxyproline measurement) in brook trout fry, 7 days after hatching. None of these effects were dose related and only at the highest dose were any deaths observed. More recently, Mayer & Mehrle (1976) showed that vitamin C levels in fish backbone also decreased after camphechlor exposure, but levels in the liver were unchanged. The authors postulated that detoxification of camphechlor required vitamin C, which moved from storage in bone to the liver. Vitamin C is involved in the conversion of proline to hydroxyproline. Competition for available vitamin C was put forward as a credible explanation for collagen synthesis effects. Camphechlor inhibited ATPase activity in trout gill microsomes at concentrations in incubates of 4 mg or more/litre (Davis et al., 1972). In channel catfish, brain and gill ATPases were more severely affected than kidney ATPase (Desaiah & Koch, 1975). Non-mitochondrial Mg-ATPase was most severely inhibited.

The acute toxicity of camphechlor for fish species is summarized in Table 4. Although the range of LC_{50} values is not great, some species differences are clear. However, the pattern of camphechlor toxicity is unrelated to fish families (Macek & McAllister, 1970). Several of the studies in Table 4 illustrate the temperature dependence of camphechlor toxicity (Hooper & Grzenda, 1955; Cope, 1965; Mahdi, 1966; Macek et al., 1969); camphechlor being more toxic at higher temperatures. No other test-condition variables showed such a clear relationship, but there was a suggestion of increased toxicity with increased alkalinity (Hooper & Grzenda, 1955; Henderson et al., 1959).

Various symptoms of camphechlor poisoning have been described for fish (Gruber, 1959; Henderson et al., 1959; Ludemann & Neumann, 1960; Workman & Neuhold, 1963; Schaper & Crowder, 1976). Initial hyperactivity is followed by muscular spasms. Later, fish show loss of equilibrium with short, jerky movements. Mosquito fish also show respiratory distress. These symptoms are similar to those caused by most chlorinated hydrocarbon insecticides. The mechanism of the toxic action of camphechlor is assumed to be mainly nervous.

There are few long-term studies on fish. Mehrle & Mayer (1975b) showed a 46% reduction in the weight of brook trout fry after 90 days' exposure to camphechlor at 0.039 µg/litre; which was the lowest concentration tested. When brook trout fry, hatched from unexposed eggs, were held in camphechlor solutions for 90 days, the mortality rate was higher than that in unexposed fry at 30 days and thereafter (Mayer et al., 1975). All fry exposed to 0.288 µg/litre died before 60 days. Yearling brook trout were less sensitive to camphechlor, showing a reduction in weight at 0.288 µg/litre and a 40% reduction at 0.502 µg/litre after exposure for 180 days. At these concentrations, length was also reduced. During 150 days of exposure to camphechlor, at concentrations ranging from 0.055 to 0.621 µg/litre, fathead minnows showed weight reductions ranging from 10.9% to 21.1%, but this was not dose-related (Mehrle & Mayer, 1975a).

Egg viability in female trout was significantly reduced when they had been exposed to camphechlor at nominal concentrations of 0.075 µg or more per litre since they were yearlings (Mayer et al., 1975). At a long-term exposure of 0.5 µg/ litre, egg viability was reduced to zero. When eggs from unexposed females were incubated in camphechlor solutions of between 0.039 to 0.502 µg/litre for 22 days, prior to hatching, they did not show any reduction in hatchability (Mayer et al., 1975; Mehrle & Mayer, 1975b).

Adaptation or resistance to camphechlor may develop, since natural populations of mosquito fish, which had either received run-off from pesticide-treated fields or been sprayed directly, were from 6 to 48 times more resistant to camphechlor than newly-exposed fish (Boyd & Ferguson, 1964).

8.2 Terrestrial Organisms

8.2.1 Insects

Several studies of the effects of technical camphechlor on honey bees gave a wide variety of results. Graves & Mackensen (1965) determined a 24-h LD_{50} at 19.08 µg/bee, whereas Torchio (1973) measured a 48-h LD_{50} as 0.144 µg/bee. In both these studies, camphechlor was applied in acetone to the dorsal thorax. Anderson & Atkins (1968) list camphechlor as "relatively non-toxic" with an LD_{50} greater than 11.0 µg/bee. Torchio (1973) looked at 3 bee species over different time periods. For honey bees and alkali bees, the numbers of deaths increased 24 - 48 h after application, but no further deaths occurred between 48 and 72 h. All bees surviving up to 72 h also survived up to 96 h. For the leaf cutting bee, there were more deaths between 48 and 72 h, but none between 72 and 96 h. Exposure of western yellowjacket wasps to the topical application of 1 µlitre drops of camphechlor resulted in mortality rates in 48 h of: 13% with exposure to 1 g/litre, 40% with exposure to 5 g/litre, and 65% with exposure to 10 g/litre (Johansen & Davis, 1972). Extensive research has been carried out on target and non-target insects. This has been reviewed by the US EPA (1979), who concluded that technical camphechlor was roughly equally toxic for both pest and beneficial insects. Lepidopterans were more resistant, possibly reflecting the long usage of camphechlor to control lepidopteran pests and the consequent development of resistance.

8.2.2 Birds

The acute toxicity of technical camphechlor for birds is summarized in Table 6. There is some species variability; sharp-tailed grouse, the most sensitive species, having an LD_{50} of 10 - 20 mg/kg body weight, and mourning dove, the least sensitive species, having an LD_{50} of 200 - 250 mg/kg body weight. Dahlen & Haugen (1954) reported a lack of motor coordination preceding death in bobwhite quail. There was a clear age effect in the toxicity of camphechlor for the mallard (Hudson et al., 1972), with young birds (36 h after

Table 6. Toxicity of camphechlor for birds

Species	Age	Sex	Route[a]	Parameter	Concentration[b] (mg/kg)	Reference
Mallard	36		oral	LD_{50}	130 (80.4 - 210)	Hudson et al. (1972)
Mallard	7 days		oral	LD_{50}	30.8 (23.3 - 40.6)	Hudson et al. (1972)
Mallard	3 - 5 months		oral	LD_{50}	70.7 (37.6 - 133)	Hudson et al. (1972)
Mallard	3 - 5 months	F	oral	LD_{50}	70.7	Tucker & Crabtree (1970)
Bobwhite quail	8 weeks		oral	LD_{50}	80 - 100	Dahlen & Haugen (1954)
Bobwhite quail	3 months	M	oral	LD_{50}	85.4	Tucker & Crabtree (1970)
Mourning dove			oral	LD_{50}	200 - 250	Dahlen & Haugen (1954)
Sharp-tailed grouse	1 - 4 years	M	oral	LD_{50}	10 - 20	Tucker & Crabtree (1970)
Fulvous tree duck	3 - 6 months	M	oral	LD_{50}	99.0	Tucker & Crabtree (1970)
Lesser sandbill crane		F	oral	LD_{50}	100 - 316	Tucker & Crabtree (1970)
Pheasant	2 weeks		diet	5-day LC_{50}	500 - 550	Heath et al., (1970)[c]
Coturnix quail	2 weeks		diet	5-day LC_{50}	600 - 650	Heath et al., (1970)[c]
Bobwhite quail	chick		diet	5-day LC_{50}	834	Heath & Stickel (1965)
Mallard	duckling		diet	5-day LC_{50}	563	Heath & Stickel (1965)

[a] Oral dosing - a single dose by gelatin capsule; dietary dosing for 5 days then 3 days of uncontaminated food.
[b] Concentrations - in mg/kg body weight for oral dosing; in mg/kg diet for dietary dosing. [c] Unpublished data.

hatching) being the least sensitive. No satisfactory explanation of this phenomenon is available. Two major field studies showed that spraying with technical camphechlor could cause death in birds. Eyer et al. (1953) applied insecticide at 2.2, 4.4, 5.5, and 6.6 kg/ha and examined domestic geese of 3 varieties. No deaths resulted at the lowest application rate. Birds of 2 varieties were killed within 3 h of direct contact with 4.4 kg/ha spray but only 1 variety was killed at 5.5 kg/ha. No birds died at the highest dose rate. The inconsistency of these results was not explained, but it is clear that the compound killed birds. McEwen et al. (1972) counted wild birds on control and sprayed areas of rangeland. Spraying at 884 g/ha reduced the number of birds relative to that in the control areas and to pre-spray observations. Dead birds (5 larks, a cowbird, a killdeer, and a dove), found on the sprayed area, contained between 9.6 and 0.1 mg camphechlor residues/kg body weight. No deaths or decrease in numbers from emigration occurred until more than a week after spraying.

Long-term toxicity of camphechlor for birds is not well documented. Keith (1966) fed sardines injected with camphechlor to white pelicans, giving the birds a daily dose of 10 or 50 mg/kg diet for 3 months. The mortality rate was high in all groups, but only the higher dose resulted in definite symptoms of poisoning prior to death. At death, birds on insecticide diets had little subcutaneous and mesentery fat. Dietary dosing of 6-month-old female, ring-necked pheasants for up to 3 months at 25, 100, 200, or 300 mg/kg diet did not cause death (Genelly & Rudd, 1956a). The initial depression in body weight observed was attributed to reduced feeding. Autopsy of mature birds dosed for 74 days with 100 or 300 mg/kg diet showed vacuolation in the livers.

Two studies on various parameters related to reproductive success in birds did not show any effects at doses up to 100 mg/kg diet. Bush et al. (1977) dosed female domestic chickens from 1 day of age up to maturity with one of 4 dose levels of camphechlor, ranging from 0.5 to 100 mg/kg diet. No significant effects were found on egg production, hatchability, or fertility. Genelly & Rudd (1956b) dosed female, ring-necked pheasants with camphechlor at either 100 or 300 mg/kg diet. Significant effects were only noticed at the higher dose rate, with reductions in egg laying and hatchability. "Relative reproductive success rate", calculated on the basis of several reproductive parameters, was 70% for controls, 62% for birds given camphechlor at 100 mg/kg diet, and 46% for birds given 300 mg/kg diet. In two studies on egg hatchability (Dunachie & Fletcher, 1969; Smith et al., 1970); camphechlor was injected into hens' eggs with no consistent effects. Maximum doses given were 500 mg/kg egg weight in one study and 1.5 mg/egg in the other. Haegele &

Tucker (1974) showed that a single oral dose of technical camphechlor at 10 mg/kg body weight did not significantly alter egg shell thickness in Japanese quail. When bobwhite quail were given technical grade camphechlor at 5, 50, or 500 mg/kg in their feed for 4 months, thyroid growth was stimulated and adrenal hypertrophy occurred at all dose levels (Hurst et al., 1974). However, only the highest dose increased uptake of I^{131}. This dose also decreased body weight. It is difficult to attribute these effects to a direct thyroid lesion.

8.2.3 Wild animals

Tucker & Crabtree (1970) reported a 96-h LD_{50} for 16 to 17-month-old male mule deer of 139 - 240 mg/kg body weight, when camphechlor was administered orally as a single dose in a gelatin capsule. The effect on *in vitro* fermentation of dry matter (alfalfa hay) by inocula of rumen fluid from mule deer was investigated by Schwartz & Nagy (1974). Inhibition was found at a dose of 1000 mg camphechlor/kg dry matter. Accidental poisoning occurred in a female Bengal tiger that ate a llama calf which had been dipped in a solution of camphechlor. Symptoms included periodic convulsions and hyperreflexia to sudden auditory and visual but not to tactile stimuli (Peavy 1975).

8.2.4 Plants

Effects of camphechlor on higher plants have only been reported for crop varieties. In greenhouse studies on cotton, using a sandy or clay soil, Franco et al. (1960) found some toxicity at a dose equivalent to a field application of 72.3 kg/ha, but only with camphechlor applied as an emulsion. When applied as a powder, the insecticide was not phytotoxic for cotton plants at a dose equivalent to 101.5 kg/ha. Hagley (1965) studied the growth of seedlings of 3 vegetables, including Chinese cabbage and tomatoes, treated with camphechlor at rates of 1.57 and 15.7 kg/ha, in the greenhouse. Both levels inhibited shoot growth in Chinese cabbage. The higher dose rate affected average weekly growth in all 3 cultivars, with little root inhibition. A level of 15.7 kg/ha was toxic for tomato seedlings, with 50% dying in the second, and a further 33% in the third week of growth. Emergence, growth, yield, and chemical composition of soybeans were not affected by the application of camphechlor at 44.8 kg/ha, which was considerably higher than recommended usage level (Probst & Everly, 1957).

8.3 Microorganisms

No effects were observed on either soil bacteria or fungi when camphechlor was applied to the soil at 22.4 kg/ha, annually, for 5 years (Martin et al., 1959), or twice yearly for 3 years, at 16.8 kg/ha (Eno et al., 1964). Bollen et al. (1954) showed that camphechlor stimulated mold numbers, 10 - 20 days after field application at 11.2 kg/ha. A higher dosage of 22.4 kg/ha, after the same period, did not show any effects on fungi. Bacteria were not affected by either dosage.

In greenhouse studies on the effects of camphechlor on nodulation bacteria, doses equivalent to between 4.9 and 40.3 kg/ha did not significantly affect bacterial growth or nodulation of legumes (Elfadl & Fahmy, 1958). Treating soil with between 12.5 and 100 mg camphechlor/kg and incubating for between 1 and 16 months in a greenhouse, did not result in any measurable effects on numbers of soil bacteria or fungi, but did stimulate nitrification and carbon dioxide evolution after one month; after 16 months, there were no effects (Eno & Everett, 1958).

The results of studies on marine and freshwater unicellular algae and protozoa are summarized in Table 7. The single study on marine algae (Ukeles, 1962) showed species variability. The dinoflagellate, Monochrysis lutheri, is the most sensitive, showing total inhibition of growth at camphechlor concentrations of 0.00015 mg/litre. The study by Stadnyk et al. (1971), whilst showing little effect on cell numbers or biomass, demonstrated marked stimulation of carbon fixation in the presence of camphechlor. At a concentration of 0.1 mg/litre, there was an initial 48% increase in carbon dioxide fixation by the green alga, Scenedesmus quadricaudata, but this became insignificant later in the 10-day exposure period. An initial increase of 450% had fallen to 30%, after 10 days' exposure to 1 mg camphechlor/litre. No explanation for this stimulation seems to be available. The complex study by O'Kelley & Deason (1976) showed that camphechlor at 0.01 mg/litre could inhibit growth in a few strains of algae (which had been isolated from the Warrior River) and stimulate growth in others. More strains showed inhibited growth at 0.1 mg/litre, but 6 out of the 21 strains used were unaffected, even by the highest dose of 1.0 mg/litre.

The lowest concentrations of camphechlor inducing toxic effects in protozoa from a salt marsh, were comparable to concentrations found in the environment (Weber et al., 1982). When a lake was treated with camphechlor (60%) at 0.1 mg/litre, protozoan numbers were reduced almost to zero (Hoffman & Olive, 1961). Turbidity of the lake water decreased until the bottom (at a depth of 4.5 m) was clearly visible.

Table 7. Toxicity of camphechlor for unicellular algae and protozoa

Organism	Temp (°C)	Sex	Sal. °/oo	Species	Exposure (days)	Concentration (mg/litre)	effect	Reference
Unicellular algae	19.5-21.5	M	22-28		10	0.00015-0.15	100% inhibition of growth	Ukeles (1962)
Blue-green alga	22	F		*Cylindrospermum licheniforme*	21	2[a]	partially toxic, reduced growth	Palmer & Maloney (1955)
Green alga	22	F		*Scenedesmus obliquus*	21	2[a]	partially toxic, reduced growth up to 14 days no effect on growth after 14 days	Palmer & Maloney (1955)
Diatom	22	F		*Gomphonema parvulum*	21	2[a]	partially toxic, reduced growth	Palmer & Maloney (1955)
Alga	20-22	F		*Selenastrum capricornutum*		0.38	EC_{50} inhibition of growth	US EPA (1980)
Green alga		F		*Scenedesmus quadricaudata*	up to 10	1.0	19% decrease in cell number, no significant effect on biomass	Stadnyk et al. (1971)
Protozoa		F		culture dominated by ciliates;(*Eupoletes* sp.) and microflagellates	1	1.3	24-h LC_{50}	Weber et al. (1982)

[a] 2 mg/litre of a 60% solution of camphechlor.
F = Freshwater.
M = Marine.

8.4 Bioaccumulation and Biomagnification

Schoettger & Olive (1961), in a study to determine the bioaccumulation of camphechlor, exposed planktonic alga (*Scenedesmus incrassatulus*) cultures to 10 µg camphechlor/litre for 384 h. The alga did not accumulate enough camphechlor to kill fish fed on it. However, periphytons (various algae, diatoms, and ciliates), exposed to the same dose of camphechlor, accumulated enough to kill fish within 24 h. Sanborn et al. (1976) reported a concentration factor of 6902 for an alga in a model ecosystem with a water concentration of 44.4 µg/litre. Concentration factors of 9600 for the snail and 890 for the mosquito were also reported.

After applying camphechlor at 50 µg/litre, to eradicate rough fish, Kallman et al. (1962) studied uptake by the rooted aquatic weed, *Potamogeton*. After 5 days and 9 days, mean concentrations in plants were 4.4 mg/kg and 14.6 mg/kg, respectively, which represents concentration factors of 4400 and 14600 over the water concentration of 1 µg/litre. Terriere et al. (1966) also found accumulation of camphechlor by aquatic plants. Plants absorbed up to 15.5 mg/kg from water containing 2 µg/litre; roots contained the highest concentrations. Salt marsh cord grass, *Spartina alterniflora*, growing near the discharge point of a camphechlor manufacturing plant, was analysed for camphechlor residues by Reimold & Durant (1972). They found maximum levels of 72.8 mg/kg in the leaves and lower concentrations in other parts of the plant. In contrast, Reimold (1974) using ^{36}Cl-labelled camphechlor, found that plant roots and rhizomes absorbed the largest amounts. The differences between uptake in these studies may be because of differences between sea water and marsh soil.

Oysters exposed to 1 µg/litre for 36 weeks bioaccumulated camphechlor throughout the pre-spawning period (Lowe et al., 1971). Concentrations in oyster tissues at 12, 24, and 36 weeks were 20 mg/kg, 23 mg/kg, and 8 mg/kg, respectively. Johnson (1966) measured camphechlor residues in plankton from Big Bear Lake, California, following 2 treatments with camphechlor at rates of 0.03 and 0.1 mg/litre, applied 2 weeks apart. Camphechlor concentrations increased to a peak of 97 mg/kg, 114 days after the final application. Concentrations decreased with time but, even 265 days after application, were still higher (at 2.0 mg/kg) than the original treatment level. Tubificid worms may accumulate camphechlor since worms collected in the Mississippi River delta contained trace amounts of camphechlor. However, worms exposed experimentally to camphechlor did not accumulate enough to kill the fish to which they were fed (Naqvi, 1973).

Fish are able to absorb and bioconcentrate significant amounts of camphechlor, a large proportion being complexed with the lipid stores. Schaper & Crowder (1976) found that exposing mosquito fish to a fatally-toxic level of 2 mg camphechlor/litre for 8 h did not result in bioconcentration, the average concentration in whole fish being 0.586 mg/kg. Thus, exposure for 8 h is not sufficient for bioaccumulation to occur in fish. When ^{14}C-labelled camphechlor was added to a terrestrial-aquatic model ecosystem at 44.4 µg/litre in the water, mosquito fish concentrated camphechlor by a factor of 4247 (Sanborn et al., 1976). Hughes (1970) exposed bluegills to 17.3 µg/litre or 70.3 µg/litre, and achieved camphechlor concentrations in the fish of 9.4 mg/kg and 7.7 mg/kg, respectively, after 96 h. Mayer et al. (1975) carried out several studies on brook trout. Brook trout fry, when exposed to camphechlor concentrations of 0.041 - 0.5 µg/litre, concentrated the chemical between 4900 and 76 000 times. Large CF values, recorded after 15 days, were partially attributed to the presence of a yolk sac, which contains large quantities of lipid. Falling values, occurring after 60 days, were due to the disappearance of the yolk sac, and the rise after 90 days to the increasing lipid content of maturing fry. Yearling brook trout bioconcentrated less camphechlor than fry during the 161-day exposure, achieving bioconcentration factors of between 3200 and 16000.

Residues of camphechlor found in fish from camphechlor-treated lakes are usually similar to levels measured in the laboratory, indicating that free-living fish can bioconcentrate camphechlor by a factor of several thousand. Kallman et al. (1962) studied the uptake of camphechlor by rainbow trout and bullhead in Clayton Lake, New Mexico, following an application of the pesticide. Seventy-two hours after treatment, the average concentration of camphechlor in the water was 2 µg/litre, and the concentration factors were 1700 for trout and 2100 for bullheads. After 5 days, the average water concentration of camphechlor was 11.5 µg/litre and, at this concentration, bullheads contained mean body residues of 13 mg/kg and were severely affected. After the water concentration stabilized at 1 µg/litre, trout exposed to this water had concentration factors ranging from 800 to 2500 after 7 days, and factors of between 1300 and 3500 after 17 days. After 108 to 170 days exposure, trout showed body residues of 0.3 mg/kg, but the water concentration had fallen to non-detectable levels.

In a similar study, Terriere et al. (1966) monitored the relationship between camphechlor levels in 2 Oregon lakes (Davis Lake treated with 80 µg camphechlor/litre and Miller Lake treated with 40 µg/litre). In Davis Lake, residues were measured in rainbow trout and Atlantic salmon; the trout consistently accumulated more camphechlor than the salmon. As in experimental exposures (Mayer et al., 1975), these fish concentrated camphechlor by a factor of several thousand. In Miller Lake, where the water concentration of camphechlor was 0.84 (0.70 - 1.1) μg/litre, brook trout, the only species monitored in this lake, concentrated camphechlor 14 800 times.

Hughes & Lee (1973) found that predator fish accumulated less camphechlor than prey fish. Bluegills and suckers, both prey fish, accumulated whole body residues of 9.4 mg/kg and 10.6 mg/kg, respectively, whereas predator fish, i.e., bass, northern pike, and walleyes, accumulated residues of only 2.2, 3.3, and 1.2 mg/kg, respectively. This suggests that the biomagnification of camphechlor in aquatic food chains may not be as great as might be indicated from bioconcentration factors.

Bioconcentration factors in a freshwater model ecosystem were shown by Metcalf (1976) to be 5 for plankton, 176 - 1152 for carp, 200 for insects, and 200 for crayfish.

There are no data on birds and mammals from which residue levels can be related to exposure levels.

8.5 Population and Community Effects

The effects of the application of 0.1 mg camphechlor/litre to control rough fish on the macroscopic bottom fauna of a lake in Colorado were studied by Cushing & Olive (1956). During the first 3 weeks following treatment, treated and control lakes were sampled fairly frequently and, thereafter, samples were taken approximately every other week. Tendipedes were killed immediately, and no larvae were found in the following 8 months. *Chaoborus* were not immediately affected, but numbers began to decline 3 months later. None were found 6 months after treatment. The authors speculated that the *Chaoborus*, which prey on tendipedes, starved to death. The number of oligochaetes increased, probably due to the extra organic matter available. In the control lake, the numbers of tendipedid, *Chaoborus*, and oligochaete remained fairly constant throughout the sampling period. *Chaoborus* numbers fell in late June/August when emergence was at its peak but, unlike the experimental lake, repopulation occurred in September.

Needham (1966) studied plankton and aquatic invertebrates in 4 North Dakota lakes. The first lake (9.7 ha, depth 2.7 m) was treated with 35 μg camphechlor/litre. Samples were taken prior to treatment and 1 week, 1 month, and 1 year after treatment. Plankton were monitored as numbers of organisms per litre. *Keratella* decreased from 91 pre-treatment to 15, one week after treatment, and subsequently to very low numbers. *Asplanchna* increased from 73 to 106, 1 week after treatment, but none were present in samples taken 1 month or 1 year later. Numbers of Daphnia decreased from 244 to 18, 1 week after treatment, increasing to 129 after 1 month but dropping to 28 after 1 year. Bosmina increased from 98 to 130 following treatment, but declined to 18 after 1 month and had only risen to 25, 1 year later. Copepoda (Diaptomus, Cyclops, and undetermined nauplii) declined in numbers after treatment, but the number of nauplii had begun to increase again, 1 year after treatment. Five invertebrate genera that lived on water plants were found in significant numbers. Gammarus varied throughout the study but remained abundant. Callibaetis, Caenis, and Ischnura decreased 1 week and 1 month after treatment, but were more abundant after 1 year. Tendipes decreased from 44 (prior to treatment) to 9, 1 week after treatment, increasing to 48, 1 month after treatment and falling back to 25, 1 year after treatment. Gastropoda (Physa and Gyraulus) increased from 771 before treatment to 1107, 1 week, 1366, 1 month, and 1558, 1 year after treatment. In the lake bottom fauna, only 2 genera were abundant; Gammarus, which fluctuated greatly during the study and tendipedes, which decreased following treatment but, 1 year later, had increased again to original numbers in samples. Comparison between plant-inhabiting organisms and bottom fauna did not reveal any shifting of populations, 1 year after treatment, apart from Physa, which increased greatly.

The second lake studied by Needham (1966) (having a surface area of 6 ha and a maximum depth of 5.5 m) was treated twice with camphechlor, first with 25 μg/litre and then, 53 days later, with 90 μg/litre. Samples were taken 1 day before, and 11, 33, and 371 days after the initial treatment. Plankton were monitored as numbers of organisms per litre. A decline in population was recorded for all genera found in significant numbers. Brachionus, which had decreased from 114 to 108 organisms/litre, 11 days after treatment, decreased to 15 after 33 days and to 3 after 371 days. The numbers of the other abundant rotifer, Asplanchna increased from 24 to 194, 11 days after treament but dropped after 33 days to 16; by 371 days, there was only one organism/litre. Daphnia, Ceriodaphnia, and Bosmina were the most abundant zooplankton. Both Daphnia and Ceriodaphnia showed similar patterns, an increase in numbers, 11 days after treatment, and a subsequent decline. Bosmina had declined from 314 to 283, 11 days after treatment, and continued to decline reaching 50 after 33 days; none were found in the 371-day sample. Copepods also decreased in numbers during the study. Although the number of Cyclops had increased between 11 and 33 days, it decreased again after 371 days.

The third lake studied by Needham (1966) (a glacial lake of 370 ha and an average depth of 2.7 m) was treated with

10 µg camphechlor/litre followed 2 days later by 5 µg/litre, and a fourth lake (40.5 ha, maximum depth 4.9 m) was treated with 5 µg/litre. Results from this lake were similar to those from the second; camphechlor failed to affect any of the organisms sampled.

When sediments containing camphechlor were disturbed by dredging, camphechlor was released into the water leading to higher concentrations in aquatic flora and fauna, but this did not appear to affect the biological balance in the area (Reimold & Durant, 1974).

8.6 Effects on the Abiotic Environment

Five annual field applications of 22.4 kg camphechlor/ha did not have any effect on the moisture content, total infiltration, and aggregation of the soil (Martin et al., 1959).

9. PREVIOUS EVALUATIONS OF CAMPHECHLOR BY INTERNATIONAL BODIES

Camphechlor was evaluated by the Joint Meeting on Pesticide Residues (JMPR) in 1968 and 1973 (FAO/WHO, 1969, 1974). In 1968, no recommendations were made because of the many unresolved questions. In 1973, the meeting concluded that it could not establish an ADI for a material that varied in composition according to the method of manufacture.

IARC (1979) evaluated the carcinogenic hazard resulting from exposure to camphechlor and concluded that "there is sufficient evidence that toxaphene is carcinogenic in mice and rats. In the absence of adequate data in humans, it is reasonable, for practical purposes, to regard toxaphene as if it presented a carcinogenic risk to humans".

Practical advice has been issued by WHO/FAO (1975) in the "Data Sheets on Pesticides", No. 20, which deals with camphechlor, and includes information on labelling, safe-handling, transport, storage, disposal, decontamination, selection, training and medical supervision of workers, first aid, and medical treatment.

Over recent years, a number of official registrations for the use of camphechlor have been drawn in several countries, for various reasons. Further details may be obtained from IRPTC.

Regulatory standards established by national bodies in 12 different countries (Argentina, Brazil, Czechoslovakia, the Federal Republic of Germany, India, Japan, Kenya, Mexico, Sweden, the United Kingdom, the USA, and the USSR) and the EEC can be obtained from the IRPTC (International Register of Potentially Toxic Chemicals) Legal File (IRPTC, 1983).

IPRTC (1983), in its series "Scientific reviews of Soviet literature on toxicity and hazards of chemicals", issued a review on camphechlor.

10. EVALUATION OF HUMAN HEALTH RISKS AND EFFECTS ON THE ENVIRONMENT

10.1 Camphechlor Toxicity

The acute toxicity of camphechlor in the rat is moderate, i.e., the oral LD_{50} ranges from 60 to 120 mg/kg body weight. Camphechlor is readily absorbed via all routes of entry. It is metabolized in the body, but a certain amount of accumulation in adipose tissue takes place on continuous exposure.

Signs and symptoms of poisoning are salivation and vomiting and, at higher exposures, excitation of the CNS with convulsions, respiratory failure, and death. On prolonged exposure of animals, hypertrophy of the liver with induction of microsomal enzymes (5 mg/kg in the diet or 0.25 mg/kg body weight per day) are the major findings.

Camphechlor has been shown not to have an effect on reproduction and it is not teratogenic. It is mutagenic in a bacterial test, but the results of a dominant lethal test in mice were negative. There is sufficient evidence for its carcinogenicity for rats and mice. Epidemiological studies are inadequate to evaluate the carcinogenic potential of camphechlor for human beings.

10.2 Exposure to Camphechlor

Exposure of the general population is mainly through residues in food. However, these are normally below residue tolerances. Accidental over-exposure has occurred as a result of contamination of food with camphechlor.

In the past, occupational exposure to camphechlor may occasionally have been considerable. Nevertheless, only a few cases of adverse effects have been reported. Workplace exposures above the permissible level have been reported.

10.3 Effects on the Environment

Movement of camphechlor through the environment is not clearly understood, but the dominant factor in the distribution of the chemical appears to be its high volatility. Camphechlor is a widespread contaminant of aquatic ecosystems. Residues have also been found in non-aquatic organisms.

Camphechlor has been used extensively as a fish poison to clear rough fish from lakes before introducing game fish. The toxic effects have not only been directly on adult fish but also, via adult females, on the development of eggs and young. Non-target aquatic organisms havere also been affected. Some invertebrates showed long-term deleterious effects of camphechlor poisoning. The environmental levels of camphechlor in waters where the chemical has not been deliberately applied can exceed laboratory concentrations that have caused death or sublethal lesions in experimental fauna. Thus, camphechlor presents a major hazard for aquatic organisms.

Available field data suggest that birds have been adversely affected by camphechlor.

10.4 Conclusions

1. Although no serious adverse effects on workers resulting from occupational exposure to camphechlor have been reported, and epidemiological studies remain inadequate, this chemical should be considered for practical purposes as being potentially carcinogenic for human beings.

2. For the same reason, and recognizing the limitations of residue analysis for camphechlor, as well as the reluctance of the JMPR to issue an ADI, reservations must remain about the safety of this chemical in food, despite the relatively low residues so far reported.

3. Environmentally, camphechlor is a major hazard for aquatic and also some terrestrial species.

4. Taking into account these considerations, it is felt that the use of this chemical should be discouraged, except where there is no adequate alternative.

REFERENCES

ALBAUGH, D.W. (1972) Insecticide tolerances of two crayfish populations Procambarus actus in South-Central Texas. Bull. env. Contam. Toxicol., 8: 334-338.

ALEXANDER, M. (1965) Persistence of chlorinated hydrocarbon insecticides in soils. Soil Sci. Soc. Am. Proc., 29: 1-7.

ANDERSON, L.D. & ATKINS, E.L. (1968) Pesticide usage in relation to beekeeping. Annu. Rev. Entomol., 13: 213-238.

ARSCOTT, G.H., MICHENER, S., & BILLS, D.D. (1976) Effect of toxaphene on the performance of white leghorn layers and their progeny. Poult. Sci., 55: 1130-1131.

ASHIROVA, S.A. (1971) Work hygiene and effectiveness of health measures in the manufacture of chlorinated terpenes. Nauch. Tr. Leningrad Gos. Instit. Usoversh. Vrachei, 98: 26-30 (in Russian; Chem. Abstr., 79: 13949).

BADAEVA, L.N. (1976) The effect of polychlorocamphene on some organs and their nervous apparatus in pregnant animals. Bull. exp. Biol. Med., 82: 945-947.

BOLLEN, W.B., MORRISON, H.E., & CROWELL, H.H. (1954) Effect of field treatments of insecticides on number of bacteria, Streptomyces, and molds in soil. J. econ. Entomol., 47: 302-306.

BOYD, C.E. & FERGUSON, D.E. (1964) Susceptibility and resistance of mosquito fish to several insecticides. J. econ. Entomol., 57: 430-431.

BOYD, E.M. (1972) Protein deficiency and pesticide toxicity, Springfield, Illinois, Charles C. Thomas Publishing Company, p. 231.

BRADLEY, J.R., SHEETS, T.J., & JACKSON, M.D. (1972) DDT and toxaphene movement in surface water from cotton plots. Environ. Qual. Saf., 1: 102-105.

BURKE, W.D. & FERGUSON, D.E. (1969) Toxicities of four insecticides to resistant and susceptible mosquito fish in static and flowing solutions. Mosq. News, 29: 96-101.

BUSH, P.B., KIKER, J.T., PAGE, R.K., BOOTH, N.H., & FLETCHER, O.J. (1977) Effects of graded levels of toxaphene on poultry residue accumulation, egg production, shell quality and hatchability in white leghorns. J. agric. food Chem., 25: 928-932.

BUTLER, P.A. (1962) Effects on commercial fisheries, Washington DC, US Department of the Interior, Fish and Wildlife Service (Circular No. 143).

BUTLER, P.A. (1963) Commercial fisheries investigations, pesticide-wildlife studies: a review of Fish and Wildlife Service investigations during 1961 and 1962, Washington DC, US Department of the Interior, Fish and Wildlife Service, p. 11 (Circular No. 167).

BUTLER, P.A. (1964) Pesticide-wildlife studies 1963: a review of Fish and Wildlife Service investigations during the calendar year, Washington DC, US Department of the Interior, Fish and Wildlife Service, p. 5 (Circular No. 199).

BUTLER, P.A., WILSON, A.J., & RICK, A.J. (1962) Effects of pesticides on oysters. Proc. Natl Shellfisheries Assoc., 51: 23-32.

CANADA, DEPARTMENT OF NATIONAL HEALTH AND WELFARE (1978) Guidelines for Canadian drinking water quality, Ottawa, Department of National Health and Welfare.

CAREY, A.E., WIERSMA, G.B., & TAI, H. (1976) Pesticide residues in urban soils from 14 United States cities, 1970. Pestic. Monit. J., 10: 54-60.

CASIDA, J.E., HOLMSTEAD, R.L., KHALIFA, S., KNOX, J.R., OHSAWA, T., PALMER, K.J., & WONG, R.Y. (1974) Toxaphene insecticide: A complex biodegradable mixture. Science, 183: 520-521.

CHAIYARACH, S., RATANANUN, V., & HARREL, R.C. (1975) Acute toxicity of the insecticides toxaphene and carbaryl and the herbicides propanil and molinate to four species of aquatic organisms. Bull. environ. Contam. Toxicol., 14: 281-284.

CHERNOFF, N. & CARVER, B.D. (1976) Fetal toxicity of toxaphene in rats and mice. Bull. environ. Contam. Toxicol., 15: 660-664.

CHANDURKAR, P.S. & MATSUMURA, F. (1979) Metabolism of toxicant B and toxicant C of toxaphene in rats. Bull. environ. Contam. Toxicol., 21: 539-547.

CLAYBORN, H.V., MANN, H.D., IVEY, M.C., REDELEFF, R.D., & WOODARD, G.T. (1963) Excretion of toxaphene and strobane in the milk of dairy cows. J. agric. food Chem., 11: 286-289.

CLAPP, K.L., NELSON, D.M., BALL, J.T., & ROUSEK, E.J. (1971) Effects of toxaphene on the hepatic cells of rats. Proc. Ann. Meeting W. Section Am. Soc. Animal Sci., 22: 313-323.

COFFIN, D.E. & McCLEOD, H.A. (1975) Current pesticide residue status of Canadian diets and adipose tissue. In: Seventh Eastern Canada Symposium on Pesticide Residue Analysis Proceedings, Toronto, May 20-23.

CONLEY, B.E. (1952) Pharmacological properties of toxaphene, a chlorinated hydrocarbon insecticide. J. Am. Med. Assoc., 149: 1135-1137.

COPE, O.B. (1965) Sport Fishery Investigations. In: The effect of pesticides on fish and wildlife, Washington DC, US Department of the Interior, Fish and Wildlife Service, pp. 51-64 (Circular No. 226).

COURTENAY, W.R. & ROBERTS, M.H. (1973) Environmental effects on toxaphene toxicity to selected fishes and crustaceans, Washington DC, US Environmental Protection Agency, 73 pp (US EPA Report EPA/R3-73-035).

CROWDER, L.A. & DINDAL, E.F. (1974) Fat of ^{36}Cl-toxaphene in rats. Bull. environ. Contam. Toxicol., 12: 320-327.

CUSHING, C.E., & OLIVE, J.R. (1956) Effects of toxaphene and rotenone upon macroscopic bottom fauna of two Northern Colorado reservoirs. Trans. Am. Fish. Soc., 86: 294-301.

DAHLEN, J.H. & HAUGEN, A.O. (1954) Acute toxicity of certain insecticides to the bobwhite quail and mourning dove. J. Wildl., 18: 477-481.

DAVIS, P.W., FRIEDHOFF, J.M., & WEDEMEYER, E.A. (1972) Organochlorine insecticide, herbicide and polychlorinated biphenyl (PCB) inhibition of $Na^{+}K^{+}$-ATPase in rainbow trout Bull. environ. Contam. Toxicol., 8: 69-72.

DEICHMANN, W.B., ed. (1973) The chronic toxicity of organochlorine pesticides in man. In: Deichmann, W.B., ed. Pesticides and the environment: selected papers presented at the 8th International American Conference on Toxicology and Occupational Medicine, University of Miami, Miami, Florida, July, 1973, pp. 347-420.

DESAIAH, D. & KOCH, R.B. (1975) Toxaphene inhibition of ATPase activity in catfish, Ictalurus punctatus tissues. Bull. environ. Contam. Toxicol., 13: 238-244.

DESAIAH, D., MEHROTA, B.D., KINZEY, R., & TROTTMAN, C.H. (1979) Effects of toxaphene, kepone and mirex on key gluconeogenic enzymes in rat liver. Fed. Proc., 8: 538.

DOMANSKI, J.J., HAIRE, P.L., & SHEETS, T.J. (1974) Insecticide residues on 1973 US tobacco products. Tobacco Sci., 18: 108-109.

DOMANSKI, J.J. & GUTHRIE, F.E. (1974) Pesticide residues in 1972 cigars. Bull. environ. Contam. Toxicol., 11: 312-314.

DOMANSKI, J.J. & SHEETS, T.J. (1973) Insecticide residues on 1970 US auction market tobacco. Tobacco, 175: 29.

DUNACHIE, J.F. & FLETCHER, W.W. (1969) An investigation of the toxicity of insecticides to birds eggs using the egg-injection technique. Ann. appl. Biol., 64: 409-423.

DURANT, C.J. & REIMOLD, R.J. (1972) Effects of estuarine dredging of toxaphene-contaminated sediments in Terry Creek, Brunswick, Georgia, 1971. Pestic. Monit. J., 6: 94-96.

ELFADL, M.A. & FAHMY, M. (1958) Effect of DDT, BHC, and toxaphene on nodulation of legumes and soil microorganisms. Agric. Res. Rev., 36: 339-350.

EMBRY, T.L. (1972) Search for abnormalities of heme synthesis and sympathoadrenal activity in workers regularly exposed to pesticides. Tex. Rep. Biol. Med., 30: 203.

ENO, C.F. & EVERETT, P.H. (1958) Effects of soil applications of 10 chlorinated hydrocarbon insecticides on soil microorganisms and the growth of stringless Black Valentine beans. Proc. Soil Sci. Soc. Am., 22: 235-238.

ENO, C.F., WILSON, J.W., CHILSHOLM, R.D., & KOBLITSKY, L. (1964) The effect of soil applications of six chlorinated hydrocarbon insecticides on vegetable crops and soil microorganisms. Proc. Florida State Hort. Soc., 77: 223-229.

EPSTEIN, S.S., ARNOLD, E., ANDREA, J., BASS, W., & BISHOP, Y. (1972) Detection of chemical mutagens by the dominant lethal assay in the mouse. Toxicol. appl. Pharmacol., 23: 288-335.

EYER, J.R., FALKNER, L.R., & MCCARTY, R.T. (1953) Effect of toxaphene and DDT on geese in cotton fields. New Mexico Agric. Exp. Sta., Bull., 1078: 1-6.

FAO/WHO (1969) Toxaphene. In: 1968 evaluations of some pesticide residues in food, pp. 267-283.

FAO/WHO (1974) Camphechlor. In: 1973 evaluations of some pesticide residues in food, pp. 92-118.

FATTAH, I.C.M.A. & CROWDER, L.A. (1980) Plasmamembrane ATPC-ases from various tissues of the cockroach (Periplanita americana) and mouse influenced by toxaphene. Bull. environ. Contam. Toxicol., 24: 356-363.

FERGUSON, D.E., CULLEY, D.D., COTTON, W.D., & DODDS, R.P. (1964) Resistance to chlorinated hydrocarbon insecticides in three species of freshwater fish. Bioscience, 14: 43-44.

FERGUSON, D.E., CULLEY, D.D., & COTTON, W.D. (1965) Tolerances of two populations of fresh water shrimp to five chlorinated hydrocarbon insecticides. J. Miss. Acad. Sci., 11: 235-237.

FITZHUGH, O.G. & NELSON, A.A. (1951) Comparison of chronic effects produced in rats by several chlorinated hydrocarbon insecticides. Fed. Proc., 10: 295.

FRANCO, C.M., FRAGA, C.C., & NEVES, O.S. (1960) [Effects of the addition of insecticides to the soil on the development of cotton crops.] Bragantia, 19: 13-25 (in Portugese).

GAINES, T.B. (1969) Acute toxicity of pesticides. Toxicol. appl. Pharmacol., 14: 5-534.

GENELLY, R.E. & RUDD, R.L. (1956a) Chronic toxicity of DDT, Toxaphene and Dieldrin to ring-necked pheasants. Calif. Fish Game, 42: 5-14.

GENELLY, R.E. & RUDD, R.L. (1956b) Effects of DDT, Toxaphene and Dieldrin on pheasant reproduction. AUK, 73: 529-539.

GLEASON, M.N., GOSSELIN, R.E., HODGE, H.C., & SMITH, R.P., ed. (1969) Clinical toxicology of commercial products - acute poisoning, 3rd ed., Baltimore Maryland, Williams and Wilkins Company, Section II, Ingredients Index.

GOSSELIN, R.E., HODGE, H.C., SMITH, R.P., & GLEASON, M.N. (1976) Clinical toxicology of commercial products, Baltimore, Maryland, Williams and Wilkins Company, p. 189.

GRAVES, J.B. & MACKENSEN, O. (1965) Topical application and insecticide resistance studies on the honey bee. J. econ. Entomol., 58: 990-993.

GRIFFIN, D.E. & HILL, W.E. (1978) In vitro breakage of plasmid DNA by mutagens and pesticides. Mutat. Res., 52: 161-169.

GRUBER, R. (1959) Toxicité pour Tilapia melanopleura de deux insecticides: l'Endrine et la Toxaphene. Bull. Agr. Congo Belge, 50: 131-139.

GUYER, G.E., ADKISSON, P.L., DUBOIS, K., MENZIE, C., NICHOLSON, H.P., ZWEIG, G., & DUNN, C.L. (1971) Toxaphene status report. Special report to Hazardous Materials Advisory Committee, Washington DC, US Environmental Protection Agency.

HAEGELE, M.A. & TUCKER, R.K. (1974) Effects of 15 common environmental pollutatnt on eggshell thickness in mallards and coturnix. Bull. environ. Contam. Toxicol., 11: 98-102.

HAGLEY, E.A.C. (1965) Effects of insecticides on the growth of vegetable seedlings. J. econ. Entom., 58: 777-778.

HARRIS, R.L. & JONES, R.H. (1962) Larvicide tests with colony-reared Culicoides variipennis. J. econ. Entomol., 55: 575-576.

HAUN, E.C. & CUETO, C. (1967) Fatal toxaphene poisoning in a 9-month-old infant. Am. J. Dis. Child, 113: 616-618.

HEATH, R.G. & STICKEL, L.F. (1965) Protocol for testing the acute and relative toxicity of pesticides to penned birds, Washington DC, US Department of the Interior, US Fish and Wildlife Service, pp. 18-24 (Circular No. 226).

HENDERSON, C.F., PICKERING, Q.H., & TARZWELL, C.M. (1959) Relative toxicity of ten chlorinated hydrocarbon insecticides to four species of fish. Trans. Am. Fish. Soc., 88: 23-32.

HOFFMAN, D.A. & OLIVE, J.R. (1961) The effects of rotenone and toxaphene upon plankton of two Colorado reservoirs. Limnol. Oceanogr., 6: 219-222.

HOLMSTEAD, R.L., KHALIFA, S., & CASIDA, J.E. (1974) Toxaphene composition analyzed by combined gas chromatography-chemical ionization mass spectrometry. J. agric. food Chem., 22: 939-944.

HOOPER, F.F. & GRZENDA, A.R. (1955) The use of toxaphene as a fish poison. Trans. Am. Fish Soc., 85: 180-190.

HOOPER, N.K., AMES, B.N., BALEK, M.A., & CASIDA, J.E. (1979) Toxaphene, a complex mixture of polychloroterpenes and a major insecticide, is mutagenic. Science, 205: 591-593.

HUDSON, R.H., TUCKER, R.K., & HAEGALE, M.A. (1972) Effect of age on sensitivity. Acute oral toxicity of 14 pesticides to mallard ducks of several ages. Toxicol. appl. Pharmacol., 22: 556-561.

HUGHES, R. (1970) Studies on the persistence of toxaphene in treated lakes, PhD thesis, Ann Arbor, Michigan, Xerox University Microfilms, pp 7-24, 751.

HUGHES, R.A. & LEE, G.F. (1973) Toxaphene accumulation in fish in lakes treated for rough fish control. Environ. Sci. Technol., 7: 934-939.

HURST, J.G., NEWCOMER, W.S., & MORRISON, J.A. (1974) Some effects of DDT, toxaphene and polychlorinated biphenyl on thyroid function in bobwhite quail. Poult. Sci., 53: 125-133.

IARC (1979) Some halogenated hydrocarbons, Lyons, International Agency for Research on Cancer, pp. 327-348 (Monographs on the Evaluation of the Carcinogenic Risk of Chemicals to Humans, Vol. 20).

IRPTC (1983a) Toxaphene. IRPTC Bull., 5: 27-28.

IRPTC (1983b) Scientific reviews of Soviet literature on toxicity and hazards of chemicals, Toxaphene, Moscow, Centre of International Projects (GKNT, No. 32).

IRPTC (1983c) Legal file, Vols. 1 & 2, Geneva, International Register of Potentially Toxic Chemicals, United Nations Environment Programme.

JEFFERY, W.H., AHLIN, T.A., GOREN, C., & HARDY, W.R. (1976) Loss of warfarin effect after occupational insecticide exposure. J. Am. Med. Assoc., 236: 2881-2882.

JOHANSEN, C.A. & DAVIS, H.G. (1972) Toxicity of nine insecticides to the western yellowjacket. J. econ. Entomol., 65: 40-42.

JOHNSON, W.C. (1966) Toxaphene treatment of Big Bear Lake, California. Calif. Fish Game, 52: 173-179.

JOHNSTON, B.L. & EDEN, W.G. (1953) The toxicity of aldrin, dieldrin and toxaphene to rabbits by skin absorption. J. Econ. Entomol., 46: 702-703.

KADIS, V.W., BREITKREITZ, W.E., & JONASSON, O.J. (1970) Insecticide levels in human tissues of Alberta residents. Can. J. Public Health, 61: 413-416.

KALLMAN, B.J., COPE, O.B., & NAVARRE, R.J. (1962) Distribution and detoxication of Toxaphene in Clayton Lake, New Mexico. Trans. Am. Fish. Soc., 91: 14-22.

KATZ, M. (1961) Acute toxicity of some organic insecticides to three species of salmonids and to the three-spined stickleback. Trans. Am. Fish. Soc., 90: 264-268.

KEISER, R.K., Jr, JULIA, A.A.A., & RAFAEL, M.S. (1973) Pesticide levels in estuarine and marine fish and invertebrates from the Guatemalan Pacific Coast. Bull. Marine Sci., 23: 905-924.

KEITH, J.O. (1966) Insecticide contaminations in wetland habitats and their effects on fish-eating birds. J. appl. Ecol. Suppl., 3: 71-85.

KENNEDY, G.L., FRAWLEY, J.P., & CALANDRA, J.C. (1973) Multigeneration reproductive effects of three pesticides in rats. Toxicol. appl. Pharmacol., 25: 589-596.

KEPLINGER, M.L., DEICHMANN, W.B., & SALA, F. (1970) Effects of combinations of pesticides on reproduction in mice. In: Inter-American Conference on Toxicology and Occupational Medicine. Pesticide Symposia, pp. 125-138.

KINOSHITA, F.K., FRAWLEY, J.P., & DUBOIS, K.P. (1966) Quantitative measurement of induction of hepatic microsomal enzymes by various dietary levels of DDT and toxaphene in rats. Toxicol. appl. Pharmacol., 9: 505-513.

KORN, S. & EARNEST, R. (1974) Acute toxicity of twenty insecticides to striped bass Morone saxatilis. Calif. Fish Game, 60: 128.

KUZMINSKAYA, U.A. & IVANITSKI, I.V.A. (1979) Study of some biological indices of the state of the sympathoadrenaline system under the effect of polychlorocampher. Environ. Health Perspect., 30: 91-95.

LACKEY, R.W. (1949) Observations on the acute and chronic toxicity of toxaphene in the dog. J. ind. Hyg. Toxicol., 3: 117-120.

LAFLEUR, K.S., WOJECK, G.A., & MCCASKILL, W.R. (1973) Movement of toxaphene and fluoneturon through Dunbar soil to underlying ground water. J. environ. Qual., 2: 515-518.

LEHMAN, A.J. (1952a) Chemicals in foods: A report to the Association of Food & Drug Officials on current developments. Part II. Pesticides Section II. Dermal Toxicity. Assoc. Food Drug Offic. US, Q. Bull., 16: 3-9.

LEHMAN, A.J. (1952b) A report to the Association of Food & Drug Officials on current developments. Section III. Subacute and chronic toxicity. Assoc. Food Drug Offic. US, Q. Bull., 16: 47-53.

LOWE, J.I. (1964) Chronic exposure of spot, Leiostomus xanthurus, to sublethal concentrations of toxaphene in sea water. Trans. Am. Fish. Soc., 93: 396-399.

LOWE, J.I., WILSON, P.D., RICK, A.J., & WILSON, A.J. (1971) Chronic exposure of oysters to DDT, toxaphene, and parathion. Proc. Natl Shellfisheries Assoc., 61: 71-79.

LUEDEMANN, D. & NEUMANN, H. (1960) [Acute toxicity tests with new contact insecticides in young carp (Cyprinus carpio L.).] Z. Angew. Zool., 47: 11-33 (in German).

LUKE, M.A., FROBERG, J.E., & MASUMOTO, H.T. (1975) Extraction and clean-up of organochlorine, organophosphate, organo-nitrogen, and hydrocarbon pesticides in produce for determination by gas-liquid chromatography. J. Assoc. Offic. Anal. Chem., 58: 1020-1026.

MACEK, K.J. & McALLISTER, W.A. (1970) Insecticide susceptibility of some common fish family representatives. Trans. Am. Fish. Soc., 99: 20-27.

MACEK, K.J., HUTCHINSON, C., & COPE, O.B. (1969) Effects of temperature on the susceptibility of bluegills and rainbow trout to selected pesticides. Bull. environ. Contam. Toxicol., 4: 174-183.

MAHDI, M.A. (1966) Mortality of some species of fish to toxaphene at three temperatures. Invest. Fish Contr., 6: 3-10.

MANSKE, D.D. & JOHNSON, R.D. (1975) Pesticide residues in total diet samples. VIII. Pestic. Monit. J., 9: 94.

MARTIN, J.P., HARDING, R.B., CANNELL, G.H., & ANDERSON, L.D. (1959) Influence of five annual applications of organic insecticides on soil biological and physical properties. Soil Sci., 87: 334-338.

MAYER, F.L. & MEHRLE, P.M. (1976) Vitamin C distribution in channel catfish as affected by toxaphene. Toxicol. appl. Pharmacol., 37: 167-168.

MAYER, F.L., MEHRLE, P.M., & DWYER, W.P. (1975) Toxaphene effects on reproduction, growth and mortality of brook trout, Washington DC, US Environmental Protection Agency, Office of Research and Development, 43 pp (US EPA 600/3-75-013).

MCEWEN, L.C., KNITTLE, C.E., & RICHMOND, M.L. (1972) Wildlife effects from grasshopper insecticides sprayed on short-grass range. J. Range Manage., 25: 188-194.

MCGEE, L.C., REED, H.L., & FLEMING, J.P. (1952) Accidental poisoning by toxaphene: Review of toxicology and case reports. J. Am. Med. Assoc., 149: 1124-1126.

MEHRLE, P.M. & MAYER, F.L. (1975a) Toxaphene effects on growth and bone composition of fathead minnows, Pimephales promelas. J. Fish. Res. Board Can., 32: 593-598.

MEHRLE, P.M. & MAYER, F.L. (1975b) Toxaphene effects on growth and development of brook trout. (Salvelinus fontinalis) J. Fish. Res. Board Can., 32: 609-613.

MENZIE, C.M. (1972) Fate of pesticides in the environment. Ann. Rev. Entomol., 17: 199-222.

METCALF, R.L. (1976) Organochlorine insecticides: survey and prospects. In: Metcalf, R.L. & McKelvey, J.J., ed. Future for insecticides: needs and prospects. Advances in the environmental science and technology, Vol. 6.

MUNSON, T.O. (1976) A note on toxaphene in environmental samples from the Chesapeake Bay region. Bull. environ. Contam. Toxicol., 16: 491-494.

NAQVI, S.M. (1973) Toxicity of twenty-three insecticides to a tubificid worm Branchiura sowerbyi from the Mississippi Delta. J. econ. Entomol., 66: 70-74.

NAQVI, S.M. & FERGUSON, D.E. (1968) Pesticide tolerances of selected freshwater invertebrates. J. Miss. Acad. Sci., 14: 121-127.

NAQVI, S.M. & FERGUSON, D.E. (1970) Levels of insecticide resistance in freshwater shrimp, Palaemontes kadiakensis. Trans. Am. Fish. Soc., 99: 696-699.

NASH, R.C. & WOOLSON, E.A. (1967) Persistence of chlorinated hydrocarbon insecticides in soils. Science, 157: 728-732.

NCI (1979b) Bioassay of toxaphene for possible carcinogenicity, Cas Registry No. 8001-35-2, National Cancer Institute (Technical Report Series No. 37-1979).

NEEDHAM, R.G. (1966) Effects of toxaphene on plankton and aquatic invertebrates in North Dakota lakes, US Department of the Interior, Fish and Wildlife Service, Bureau of Sport Fishing and Wildlife (Resource Publication No. 8).

NICHOLSON, H.P., GRZENDA, A.R., LAUER, G.J., COX, W.S., & TEASLEY, J.I. (1964) Water pollution by insecticides in an agricultural river basin. I. Occurrence of insecticides in river and treated municipal water. Limnol. Oceanogr., 9: 310.

NIOSH (1977b) NIOSH manual of analytical methods Part 1. In: NIOSH monitoring methods, Vol. 1, 2nd ed., Method No. P Cam 225, Washington DC, US Department of Health, Education and Welfare, pp. 225-1-256-6 (US DHEW(NIOSH), Publication No. 77-157B).

OHSAWA, T., KNOX, J.R., KHALIFA, S., & CASIDA, J.E. (1975) Metabolic chlorination of toxaphene in rats. J. agric. food Chem., 23: 98-106.

O'KELLEY, J.C. & DEASON, T.R. (1976) Degradation of pesticides by algae, Athens, Georgia, US Environmental Protection Agency, 42 pp (Report EPA-600/3-76-022).

OLSON, K.L., MATSUMURA, F., & BOUSH, G.M. (1980) Behavioral effects on juvenile rats from perinatal exposure to low-levels of toxaphene 6, its toxic components, toxicant-A and toxicant-B. Arch. environ. Contam. Toxicol., 9: 247-257.

ORTEGA, P., HAYES, W.J., & DURHAM, W.F. (1957) Pathologic changes in the liver of rats after feeding low levels of various insecticides. AMA. Arch. Pathol., 64: 614-622.

PALMER, C.M. & MALONEY, T. E. (1955) Preliminary screening for potential algicides. Ohio J. Sci., 55: 1-8.

PARDINO, R.S., HEIDKER, J.C., & PAYNE, B. (1971) The effects of some cyclodiene pesticides, benzenehexachloride and toxaphene on mitochondrial electron transport. Bull. environ. Contam. Toxicol., 6: 436-444.

PEAKALL, D.B. (1976) Effects of toxaphene on hepatic enzyme induction and circulating steriod levels in the rat. Environ. Health Perspect., 13: 117-120.

PEAKALL, D.B. (1979) Effect of toxaphene on pyruvic and lactic acid levels in the rat. Environ. Health Perspect., 30: 97-98.

PEAVY, G.M. (1975) Use of diazepam and methocarbamol in the treatment of toxaphene poisoning in a Bengal tiger. J. Am. Vet. Med. Assoc., 167: 577-578.

PENUMARTHY, L., OEHME, F.W., SPAULDING, J.E., & RADER, W.A. (1976) Toxaphene: livestock toxicity and tissue residues. Vet. Tox., 18: 60-70.

POLLOCK, G.A. & KILGORE, W.W. (1976) The metabolism of toxaphene components. Toxicol. appl. Pharmacol., 37: 138-139.

POLLOCK, G.A. & KILGORE, W.W. (1978) Toxaphene. Res. Rev., 69: 87-140.

POLLOCK, G.A. & KILGORE, W.W. (1980) Toxicities and description of some toxaphene fractions - isolation and identification of a highly toxic component. J. Toxicol. environ. Health, 6: 115-125.

POLLOCK, R.W. (1953) Toxaphene poisoning - Report of a fatal case. Northw. Med. (Seattle), 52: 293-294.

PROBST, A.H. & EVERLY, R.T. (1957) Effect of soil insecticides on emergence, growth, yield and chemical composition of soybeans. Agron. J., 49: 385-387.

REIMOLD, R.J. (1974) Toxaphene interactions in estuarine ecosystems, Springfield, Virginia, National Technical Information Service, 89 pp (COM-75-10104/8GA).

REIMOLD, R.J. & DURANT, C.J. (1972) Toxaphene levels in Georgia survey of estuaries, Georgia, Georgia Marine Science Center, University of Georgia, 51 pp (Technical Report No. 72-2).

REIMOLD, R.J. & DURANT, C.J. (1974) Toxaphene content of estuarine fauna and flora before, during and after dredging toxaphene-contaminated sediments. Pestic. Monit. J., 8: 44-49.

REUBER, M.D. (1979) Carcinogenicity of toxaphene. J. Toxicol. environ. Health, 5: 729-748.

SAMOSH, L.V. (1974) Chromosome aberrations and character of satellite associations after accidental exposure of the human body to polychlorocamphene. Toxicol. Genet., 8: 24-27.

SANBORN, J.R., METCALF, R.L., BRUCE, W.N., & LU, P-Y. (1976) The fate of chlordane and toxaphene in a terrestrial-aquatic model ecosystem. Environ. Entomol., 5: 533-538.

SANDERS, H.O. & COPE, O.B. (1966) Toxicities of several pesticides to two species of Cladocerans. Trans. Am. Fish Soc., 95: 165-169.

SCHAPER, R.A. & CROWDER, L.A. (1976) Uptake of ^{36}Cl-toxaphene in mosquito fish, Gambusia affinis. Bull. environ. Contam. Toxicol., 15: 581-587.

SCHIMMEL, S.C., PATRICK, J.N., & FORESTER, J. (1977) Uptake and toxicity of toxaphene in several estuarine organisms. Arch. environ. Contam. Toxicol., 5: 353-367.

SCHOETTGER, R.A. & OLIVE, J.R. (1961) Accumulation of Toxaphene by fish-food organisms. Limnol. Oceanogr., 6: 216-219.

SCHWARTZ, C.C. & NAVY, J.G. (1974) Pesticide effects on in vitro dry matter digestion in deer. J. Wildl. Manage., 38: 531-534.

SHELANSKI, H.A. (1947) Various untitled reports and letters submitted to Hercules Powder Co., Smith Laboratories (unpublished).

SMITH, D.C. (1971) Pesticide residues in the total diet in Canada. Pestic. Sci., 2: 92-95.

SMITH, D.C., SANDI, E., & LEDUC, R. (1972) Pesticide residues in the total diet in Canada II-1970. Pestic. Sci., 3: 207-210.

SMITH, D.C., LEDUC, R., & CHARBONNEAU, C. (1973) Pesticide residues in the total diet in Canada III-1971. Pestic. Sci., 4: 211-214.

SMITH, S.I., WEBER, C.W., & REID, B.C. (1970) The effect of injection of chlorinated hydrocarbon pesticides on hatchability of eggs. Toxicol. appl. Pharmacol., 16: 179-185.

STADNYK, L., CAMPBELL, R.S., & JOHNSON, B.T. (1971) Pesticide effect on growth and ^{14}C assimilation in a freshwater alga. Bull. environ. Contam. Toxicol., 6: 1-8.

STALLING, D.L. & HUCKINS, J.N. (1976) Analysis and GC-MS characterization of toxaphene in fish and water, Washington DC, US Environmental Protection Agency (US EPA 600/3-76-076).

STANLEY, C.W., BARNEY, J.E., II, HELTON, M.R., & YOBS, A.R. (1971) Measurement of atmospheric levels of pesticides. Environ. Sci. Technol., 5: 430-435.

TAYLOR, J.R., CALABRESE, V.P., & BLANKE, R.V. (1979) Organochlorine and other insecticides. In: Vinken, P.J. & Bruyn, G.W., ed. Handbook of clinical neurology, Vol. 36 Intoxications of the nervous system, Part. 1, Amsterdam, New York, Elsevier/North-Holland Biomedical Press.

TERRIERE, L.C. & INGALSBE, D.W. (1953) Translocation and residual action of soil insecticides. J. econ. Entomol., 46: 751.

TERRIERE, L.C., KIIGEMAGI, U., GERLACK, A.R., & BOROVICKA, R.L. (1966) The persistence of Toxaphene in lake water and its uptake by aquatic plants and animals. J. agric. food Chem., 14: 66-69.

TEWARI, S.N. & SHARMA, I.C. (1977) Isolation and determination of chlorinated organic pesticides by thin-layer chromatography and the application to toxicological analysis. J. Chromatogr., 131: 275-284.

TORCHIO, P.F. (1973) Relative toxicity of insecticides to the honey bee, alkali bee and alfalfa leafcutting bee (Hymenoptera, Apidae, Halictidae, Megachilidae). J. Kans. Entomol. Soc., 46: 446-453.

TREON, J.F., CLEVELAND, F.P., POYNTER, B., WAGNER, B., & GAHEGAN, T. (1952) The physiologic effects of feeding experimental animals on diets containing toxaphene in various concentrations over prolonged periods, Kettering Laboratory (unpublished report).

TROTTMAN, C.H. & DESAIAH, D. (1980) Induction of rat hepatic microsomal enzymes by toxaphene pretreatment. J. environ. Sci. Health (Part B: Pesticides, food Contam. agric. Wastes), 15: 121-134.

TUCKER, R.K. & CRABTREE, D.G. (1970) Handbook of toxicity of pesticides to wildlife, US Department of the Interior, Fish and Wildlife Service, Bureau for Sport Fishing and Wildlife, pp. 116-117 (Resource Publication No. 84).

UKELES, R. (1962) Growth of pure cultures of marine phytoplankton in the presence of toxicants. Appl. Microbiol., 10: 532-537.

US EPA (1976a) Criteria document for toxaphene. Fed. Reg., 440: 9-76-014.

US EPA (1976b) Economic assessment of proposed toxic pollutant standards for manufacturers and formulators of aldrin/dieldrin, endrin, DDT and toxaphene, Washington DC, US Environmental Protection Agency (Prepared by Arthur D. Little Inc. for Environmental Protection Agency) (US EPA 230/3-76-016).

US EPA (1979) Reviews of the environmental effects of pollutants. X. Toxaphene, Washington DC, US Environmental Protection Agency (US EPA Report 600/1-79-044).

US EPA (1980) Ambient water quality criteria for toxaphene, Washington DC, US Environmental Protection Agency (Report US EPA 440/5-80-076).

VON RUMKER, R., LAWLESS, L., MEINER, A.F., LAWRENCE, K.A., KELSO, G.L., & HORAY, F. (1974) Production, distribution, use and environmental impact potential of selected pesticides, Kansas City, Missouri, Midwest Research Institute, pp. 1-439 (NTIS Publication No. 236).

WARRAKI, S. (1963) Respiratory hazards of chlorinated camphene. Arch. environ. Health, 1: 253-256.

WEBER, F.H., SHEA, T.B., & BERRY, E.S. (1982) Toxicity of certain insecticides to protozoa. Bull. environ. Contam. Toxicol., 28: 628-631.

WELCH, R.M., LEVIN, W., KUNTZMAN, R., JACOBSON, M., & CONNEY, A.H. (1971) Effect of halogenated hydrocarbon insecticides on the metabolism and uterotropic action of estrogens in rats and mice. Toxicol. appl. Pharmacol., 19: 234-246.

WHO/FAO (1975) Pesticide residues in food, Vol. 97, pp. 7-37 (Technical Report Series No. 574).

WIERSMA, G.B., MITCHELL, W.G., & STANFORD, C.L. (1972a) Pesticide residues in onions and soil - 1969. Pestic. Monit. J., 5: 345-347.

WIERSMA, G.B., TAI, H., & SAND, P.F. (1972b) Pesticide residues in soil from eight cities - 1969. Pestic. Monit. J., 6: 126-129.

WIERSMA, G.B., TAI, H., & SAND, P.F. (1972c) Pesticide residue levels in soils, FY 1969 - National Soils Monitoring Program. Pestic. Monit. J., 6: 194-201.

WORKMAN, G.W. & NEUHOLD, J.M. (1963) Lethal concentrations of toxaphene for goldfish, mosquito fish and rainbow trout, with notes on detoxification. Prog. Fish Cult., 25: 23-30.

YANG, H.S.C., WIERSMA, G.B., & MITCHELL, W.G. (1976) Organochlorine pesticide residues in sugarbeet pulps and molasses from 16 states, 1971. Pestic. Monit. J., 10: 41-43.

YAP, H.H., DESAIAH, D., CUTKAMP, L.K., & KOCH, R.B. (1975) In vitro inhibition of fish brain ATPase activity by cyclodiene insecticide and related compounds. Bull. environ. Contam. Toxicol., 14: 163-167.

ZAVON, M.R., TYE, R., & LATORRE, L. (1969) Chlorinated hydrocarbon insecticide content of the neonate. Ann. N.Y. Acad. Sci., 160: 196-200.

ZWEIG, G., PYE, E.L, SITLANI, R., & PEOPLES, S.A. (1963) Residues in milk from dairy cows fed low levels of toxaphene in their daily ration. J. agric. food Chem., 11: 70-72.